YOUR HEALTH IS YOUR WEALTH – BOOK ONE
PLEASE DON'T EAT THE DONUTS
A real world guide to gastrointestinal health

United States Copyright 2013 ©

ISBN: 1492164070
ISBN-13:   978 1492164074

Dalal, Akoury, M.D.
AWAREMed Health & Resource Center
4710 Oleander Drive
Myrtle Beach, SC 29577
843/213-1480
www.awaremed.com

CHAPTER ONE

WANTED: 20 Feet of Healthy Intestines

"Our minds are like our stomachs; they are whetted by the change of their food,
and variety supplies both with fresh appetites."
Marcus Fabius Quintilianus

The gastrointestinal tract is your body's first line of exposure to the outside world. When we take proper care of our bellies, we can cure almost any ailment. An inner coil of 20 feet of intestinal tissue works very hard to massage, manage and break down any food we eat; absorbing essential nutrients, vitamins and minerals plus exposing waste 24 hours a day. It's a hard job but some part of the body has got to do it.

Right from the start, let's look at what our gastrointestinal needs truly are.

BACTERIA

Usually viewed as dangerous, unpleasant, and unwanted invaders, *not all bacteria are bad.* In fact, there are more than 400 strains of bacteria that are good for your health that reside mostly in the intestinal tract. Moreover, amino acids, calcium, zinc, manganese, iron, copper, and phosphorus are all rendered more biologically useful in foods fermented with bacterial cultures. *These beneficial bacteria are most commonly known as probiotics, a word you are probably used to hearing bandied about in the media today.*

From birth, physicians typically encourage breast feeding. This is because breast milk contains living probiotics and most manufactured formulas don't contain these natural bacteria. Probiotics have been found to aid in the prevention of bacterial, viral, and fungal infections.

Therefore, throughout childhood and as an adult, it is important to maintain the proper balance of probiotic bacteria which has a cleansing effect on the body and helps us avoid disease. Without probiotics the intestinal processes that digest, absorb, and detoxify the foods we eat cannot proceed smoothly. *Twenty feet of tissue are screaming for help!*

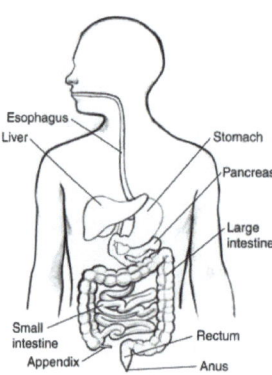

National Digestive Diseases Information Clearinghouse (NDDIC)

Improper probiotic balance can cause digestive upset from mild to severe including:

- Infant colic
- Lactose intolerance
- Yeast infections
- Antibiotic resistance
- Autoimmune disorders
- Allergies
- Ulcers
- Cancers

Imbalance occurs quickly. A good example is antibiotic use. Most patients are aware that antibiotics kill good bacteria along with the bad and this temporarily renders the body out-of-balance and susceptible to other infections or health disorders. As far as the gastrointestinal tract, overuse will disturb its entire functioning; therefore antibiotics are now prescribed much more judiciously. Another example is lactose intolerance. Most people can usually tolerate milk products better when they've been fermented because the bacteria break down lactose before the food is consumed.

Probiotics stimulate antibody production and increase the activity of white blood cells and the immune cells that target, consume, and engulf pathogens. Probiotics are also believed to reduce intestinal inflammation, which leads to the formation of the tiny "holes" in the intestinal wall that can allow large food particles into the circulation. The immune system reacts to rid the body of these foreign particles, and this state of immune reactivity can exaggerate allergic reactions to foods or environmental allergens.

One strain of yeast known as Candida albicans, is a natural resident of the digestive tract and mucus membranes throughout the body. When micro flora is abundant and the immune system is functioning well, theses yeasts are kept in check. They can quickly become overgrown when the probiotics population falls due to antibiotics or synthetic hormone use, or to an overabundance of refined carbohydrates in the diet.

Ulcers are now known to be caused by the H. pylori bacteria, which has also been linked to increases in the stomach cancer risk. When good bacteria are present in sufficient numbers, they protect the stomach lining against H. pylori. Researchers on aging are now starting to understand how a decrease in these good bacteria may be one of the reasons for the increased cancer and other illnesses as we age.

What's different today?

- Many children are born by Caesarean section and are fed formula, both of which hamper the initial development of healthy probiotic populations.
- Modern humans consume millions of times fewer Lactobacilli and other flora than our Paleolithic ancestors.
- Diets rich in refined carbohydrates and sugars enhance the growth of bad bacteria and yeasts, to the detriment of friendly bacteria.

- Diets that are heavy with meat and light on vegetables and fruits alter the activity of the friendly flora.
- Plant foods containing prebiotics (bananas, berries, asparagus, garlic, whole grains, flaxseed, tomatoes, onions, greens - especially dandelion- and legumes) are the probiotics favorite food.
- Chlorinated water has damaging effects on flora.
- The frequent use of antacids and other acid-reducing drugs lower the acidity of the gastrointestinal tract, which creates an inhospitable environment for friendly bacteria.
- Synthetic estrogens taken in the form of birth controls pills or hormone replacement also decrease micro flora populations. This is why the use of antibiotic drugs can cancel out the effects of birth control pills and cause break-through bleeding in pre-menopausal women.
- Oral steroid drugs such as Prednisone, anti-inflammatory drugs (aspirin), and inhaled steroid drugs for asthma decrease probiotic counts.
- Stress alters the balance of important hormones, and this shift can cause probiotic populations to dwindle.

ENZYMES

Our tummies also need a proper balance of enzymes that are best described as catalysts that enable our bodies to digest food, transport nutrients, carry away toxic wastes, purify blood, deliver hormones, balance cholesterol and triglycerides, nourish the brain, build protein into muscles, and feed and fortify the endocrine system. *Phew! They've got an important job to do.*

Ideally, our bodies would manufacture all the enzymes we need from food but that doesn't happen for several reasons. Most of the food we eat lacks the enzymes it would naturally contain because it's grown in nutrition-depleted soils, treated with pesticides, usually picked before it ripens (for longer shelf life), and more often than not cooked at temperatures that destroy whatever enzymes are still present. Then, the net result is that we can't utilize the nutrients.

Some of us turn to using supplements because of trouble digesting food, but it's probable that the supplements are also being poorly digested. This misconduct of poor digestion may start before you think. <u>About 30 to 40 per cent of our food should be digested in the mouth</u>. *It is recommended to chew each mouthful at least 30 times, but chewing three to five times is the actual average.* As a result, the stomach can become overworked, and to compensate other organs are enlisted in the digestion process.

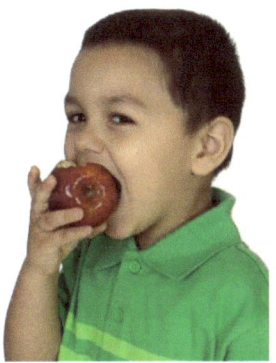

In this faulty cycle, enzymes that other organs should be using to repair tissue and maintain health, known as the systemic enzymes, are used up in the body's effort to digest food. And such a malfunctioning system might create havoc by undigested materials from food seeping into the blood stream, and the body may have allergic reactions.

Symptoms of digestive enzyme deficiency:

- Indigestion
- Gas
- Diarrhea
- Intestinal pain.
- Irregular bowel movements
- Nausea
- Heartburn
- Bloating
- Food cravings
- Food sensitivities.

In addition, this cycle can cause other conditions not normally associated with digestive problems. Underlying all these symptoms is reduced energy; from tiredness after a meal, to ever-present fatigue. Simply put: *The lack of enzymes makes the process of digestion stressful.*

Finally, many strains of probiotics produce enzymes within the gastrointestinal tract. These enzymes help to break down the foods we eat more completely. The nutrients from these foods can be better absorbed as well as reduce bloating and gas. Intestinal flora (good bacteria) make an important contribution to optimal nutrition by producing B-complex vitamins, short chain fatty acids, antioxidants, amino acids, and vitamin K.

CHAPTER TWO

TAMING THE BEAST

"For man, as for flower and beast and bird, the supreme triumph is to be most vividly, most perfectly alive."
D. H. Lawrence

If we are to tame our own belly of the beast, we must recognize that we can be our worst enemy when it comes to gastrointestinal health. If food can be our medicine then the kitchen is our pharmacy. *So let's talk frankly about food.*

WHAT ISN'T IN ORGANIC PRODUCE?

According to U.S. Department of Agriculture guidelines, <u>organic products</u> are certified to have been produced and processed without:

- *Synthetic herbicides or pesticides that are increasingly linked to birth defects, allergies, cancer, heart diseases, hormonal diseases and other health problems.*
- *Sewage sludge which often contains heavy metals, asbestos, industrial solvents, fungi, parasites, and viruses.*
- *Genetically modified organisms (GMOs).*

In fact, many diseases, including cancer, asthma, diabetes, and cardiovascular disease, have been attributed to this constant onslaught of chemicals and pesticides. <u>We're using 33 times more pesticides on foods than we did 50 years ago, but crop losses are 20 times higher because nearly 1,000 pests have developed resistance to these synthetic toxins.</u>

According to author and human metabolism research scientist Paula Baillie-Hamilton M.D., Ph.D.: *"Our bodies were never designed to protect themselves against this form of attack. As a result, our systems usually fail to process and remove most of these chemicals."* In the United States alone, more than one billion pounds of pesticides enter the environment annually. Alarmingly, tests conducted by the United States Department of Agriculture (USDA) find that conventionally grown produce crops contain three to nine times more multiple pesticide residues than organic fruit and vegetables. Furthermore, research at New York City's Columbia University recently found that babies of women exposed to chlorpyrifos and diazinon (pesticides widely used on fruits and vegetables) weighed significantly less at birth than other infants.

Conventional agriculture relies on monoculture - planting huge fields of a single crop. Not only does this technique deplete the soil and attract pests, but it also reduces plant diversity. Since 1900, 6,000 apple and 2,300 pear varieties have become extinct. These losses can result in generic weakness of plant species. By contrast organic farming conserves and promotes species diversity. By using natural agriculture techniques, including composting and crop rotation, organic farmers build fertile, healthy soil; and healthy soil can produce more nutrient-rich crops.

For centuries farmers and ranchers have cross bred plants or animals to increase the odds of getting more desired traits. A simple example is crossing apple varieties to assure getting sweet fruit. This is a technique that relies on reproduction to pass on genes. Sometimes these experiments work out and sometimes they don't. Breeding is a 'nothing ventured, nothing gained' situation. On the other hand *genetically modified organisms* (GMOs), or genetically engineered organisms (GEOs), are, in my opinion, extremely dangerous.

This Is How It Works

Most frequently a gene from one species is inserted into the gene sequence of a different species. It is a random insertion because we have neither the technology nor the understanding to place these genes. If the antibiotic resistant marker (ARM) gene makes the horizontal gene transfer, it could result in new and dangerous anti-biotic resistant disease. This serious risk was mentioned by the members of the British Medical Association as one of the reasons why they called for an immediate suspension on genetically engineered foods in the United Kingdom.

Testing

Dr. Arpad Putsztai, a Hungarian-born biochemist and nutritionist who spent 36 years at the Rowett Research Institute in Aberdeen, Scotland to become a world expert on plant lectins, authoring 270 papers and three books on the subject. In 1998 Pusztai publicly announced that the results of his research showed feeding genetically modified potatoes to rats had negative effects on their stomach lining and immune system.

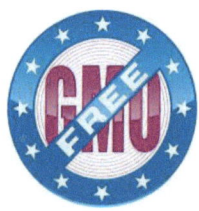

First, the nutritional content of the potatoes differed substantially from the parent line. Not only that, but also the nutritional content varied from one potato to another. This in itself invalidates U.S. Food and Drug Administration (FDA) policy, which is based on the assumption that any whole food combined with any presumed safe gene yields a safe and nutritionally stable result. Putsztai also found that rats fed a genetically modified (GM) diet in 10 days developed serious health problems such as; their white cells were sluggish, their spleen and thymus glands showed damage, and their immune systems were compromised. Some of the GM-fed rats had small, less developed brains, livers, and testicles. Others had enlarged tissues, including enlarged pancreases and intestines. After 110 days some of the changes still persisted.

The Human Effect

The GM-fed rats study time period is equivalent to about 10 human years. It's unlikely that if the same problems develop in humans, they would be traced to GM foods eaten a decade earlier. However, *at no time were U.S. citizens asked to weigh the risks of GMO's against the possible gains, yet today most of us are eating them while being kept in the dark as to the hazards we may be facing.* What we do know is that several people went into anaphylactic shock and some died from a U.S. manufacturer's GM corn. In 2001, this product from Aventis Crop Science, doing business as StarLink, was not approved for human consumption. However, it wasn't stored separately and eventually was found in tacos, tortillas, and other corn products. Over 300 items were recalled and Aventis paid out an estimated $1 billion dollars for the contamination.

At the Zoo

So it's apparent that GMO's are another significant reason to buy organically. Even animals prefer organic foods. One zoo keeper in Copenhagen noticed that chimps would eat the skin as well as the flesh of organic bananas; but if the banana wasn't organic, the chimps would peel it. Granted, it's not in everyone's budget to convert entirely to eating all organic foods, but there are some changes that are more crucial than others.

The 12 "Most-Contaminated-By-Pesticide" Fruits and Vegetables

1. APPLES
2. BELL PEPPERS
3. CELERY
4. CHERRIES
5. GRAPES
6. NECTARINES
7. PEACHES
8. PEARS
9. POTATOES
10. RASPBERRIES
11. SPINACH
12. STRAWBERRIES

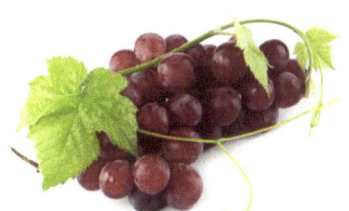

The 12 "Least-Contaminated-By-Pesticide" Fruits and Vegetables

1. ASPARAGUS
2. AVOCADOS
3. BANANAS
4. BROCCOLI
5. CAULIFLOWER
6. CORN
7. KIWIS
8. MANGOES
9. ONIONS
10. PAPAYAS
11. PINEAPPLES
12. PEAS

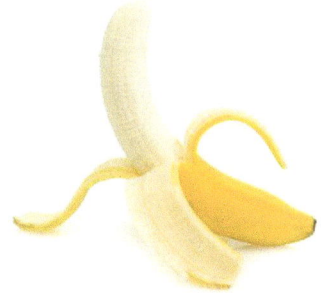

In summary, genetically modified crops are comprised of soy (81%), cotton (70%), canola (73%), corn (40%), papaya (more than 50%), zucchini, and yellow squash. *It's best to avoid them.*

WHAT ISN'T IN ORGANIC MEAT AND DAIRY?

The terminology surrounding the organic meat market can be tricky, so here are some explanations that can help you make healthier purchases for you and your family.

If it walks like a chicken and squawks like a chicken, is it good to eat? See the many differences among how healthier chickens are raised:

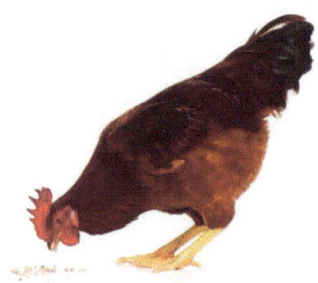

- <u>Organic chickens</u> are raised organically from birth without being fed animal byproducts, fillers such as plastic, and without antibiotics, or growth hormones added to their feed. Instead, the organic chickens are fed certified organic sprouted grains when indoors and forage when outdoors. These chicken farms are inspected and certified yearly by a third-party certification process; they must allow each bird outdoor access with at least two square feet of space to avoid overcrowding.
- <u>Free-range chickens</u> have access to outdoors most of the year by means of a fenced-in run. Each bird is required to have two square feet of space also. The feed cannot contain antibiotics or growth stimulants.
- <u>Pastured chickens</u> may be kept in cages, protected from the elements, and in order for the chickens to get new grass daily the cages are moved from one spot to the other.
- <u>Organically grown beef</u> is given access to the outdoors, fresh air, sunshine, water, and organic grass, pastureland, or feed. No confined eating is allowed and they can't be fed any animal by-products, antibiotics, or growth hormones. Organic beef takes five times as long as conventional beef to bring to the market. Organic cattle are tracked from birth to market with a paper trail that can be retraced.

Does it moo or is it good for stew? Commercial beef is also processed in many ways that can be negative to our health. Therefore, the following offers a guide to improved options:

- <u>Natural beef</u> is minimally processed and free of flavorings, colorings, chemical preservatives, and artificial or synthetic ingredients in the meat. According to the USDA, there are no regulations concerning how the natural beef was raised, fed, or processed. Producers are encouraged to communicate directly to the customers about what natural beef means. For example, some natural beef may be grown without antibiotic or growth hormones, and producers will claim such on their labels.

- <u>Grass-fed beef</u> have been allowed some pasture time, but exactly how much may vary with the producers.

One fish or two fish, these are good-to-eat fish:

- <u>Farmed fish</u> are grown in aquaculture pounds; either fresh water, as in the case of catfish, or sea water for salmon.
- <u>Wild fish</u> are caught or harvested from the wild, but are not considered organic. Wild fish are also less likely to contain pollutants such as mercury and PBCs when compared with farmed fish. The amount of omega-3 fats in fish varies greatly from 0.3 g in 3 ounces of fresh yellow-fin tuna to 0.8g in albacore tuna to 1.4 g in fresh blue-fin tuna or 0.9-1.8 in salmon. Alaskan salmon is a great health choice because they come from well-managed fisheries and cleaner waters. Sockeye salmon, keta (chum) salmon, and pink salmon (all Pacific species) are always wild.

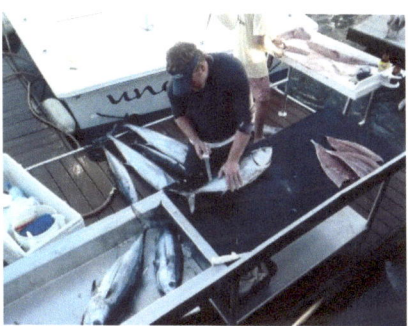

Being an omnivore isn't as easy as it used to be. The more we learn about the dangers surrounding conventional beef, the more we may consider other protein sources. But thanks to national regulations for certification, organic beef is guaranteed to be free of growth hormones, antibiotics, and animal byproducts.

Milk, milk, and milk:

There are two widely used methods to pasteurize milk. First is high temperature/short time (HTST). Milk treated this way is usually labeled "pasteurized." Second, ultra-high temperature (UHT) is usually labeled "ultra-pasteurized" and both HTST and UHT are permitted in organic production.

HTST involves holding the milk at temperatures of 161.5 degrees for at least 15 seconds and usually has a refrigerated shelf life of two to three weeks. UHT involves holding the milk at temperatures of 280 degrees for at least two seconds and has a refrigerated shelf life of two to three months. Also UTH pasteurized milk that is packaged in aseptic cartons is shelf stable and doesn't have to be refrigerated until it's opened. These procedures were designed to destroy almost all yeast, mold, and common spoilage bacteria and to ensure adequate destruction of common pathogenic heat-resistant organisms.

On the other hand, organic milk (particularly pasture-based operations) contains significantly higher levels of conjugated linoleic acid (CLA) than conventional milk. According to the American Journal of Clinical Nutrition, potential benefits of CLA include reducing the propensity to store fat, inhibiting tumor development, promoting sensitivity to insulin in the cells, increasing immune response against viral antigens, and modulating inflammatory processes. On-going studies are exploring the potential of CLA to delay the onset of type-2 diabetes, a disease reaching epidemic proportions in developed countries.

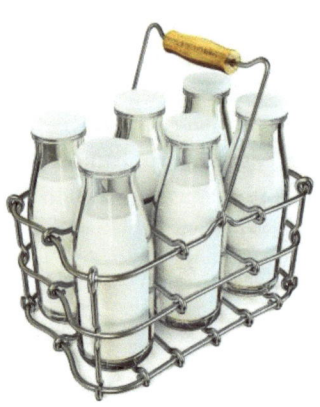

YOUR NOTES

CHAPTER THREE

DON'T HATE YOUR GUTS

"Food is an important part of a balanced diet."

Fran Lebowitz

There has been much talk of the food pyramid in recent years; how – perhaps – we've gotten it wrong putting meat in the largest tier and fruits, vegetables and grains in the smallest. I am so glad the United States Department of Agriculture has agreed with what many of us physicians and patients already knew: *Turn that pyramid upside down and reclaim your life!*

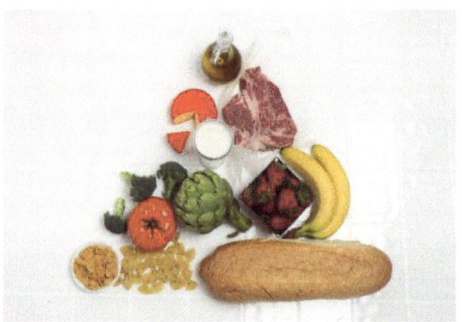

"Death begins in the colon" was the conclusion of 57 leading physicians at a symposium held at the Royal Society of Medicine of Great Britain. Their findings were that nearly <u>every known chronic disease is either directly or indirectly linked to more than 35 bacterial poisons absorbed through the intestines.</u>

Most of us don't connect headaches, depression, or heart trouble to a toxic colon (technically called alimentary toxcmia). However, the colon is a five-foot long tube that performs two primary functions – the absorption of water, electrolytes, and some vitamins; and the solidification of waste that needs to be eliminated. A healthy colon provides the body with the hydration needed to perform the myriad of functions through its absorption of water. But when a colon is toxic, its power of absorption can actually cause a condition called "auto-intoxication," or self-poisoning. Typically, this condition is linked to a poor diet and chronic constipation.

Are you constipated?

When <u>constipation</u> occurs (defined by most naturopathic physicians as less than two bowel movements a day), food transit time (the amount of time it takes for a meal to enter, and then exit the body) is greatly increased. <u>In other words, food movement in the body slows down.</u> When putrefied material stays in the colon longer than it should, the toxins have more time to enter the blood stream through the intentional cells that line the colon. This can cause a wide range of complaints, from headaches to autoimmune diseases. Additionally, slow transit time can lead to a toxic build up on the intestinal walls. This can result in reduced nutrient absorption, or mal-absorption, which deprives the body of nutrients needed to create vitality.

Moreover, scientific studies report that colon and breast cancers can be the results of years of constipation and autointoxication.

What can I do?

These compounds can help soothe and heal irritated or ulcerated gastrointestinal tissue by attaching to the site injury and protecting it from acids, bacteria, and other irritants until damage can be repaired:

- Aloe Vera Gel
- Marshmallow Root
- Slippery Elm Bark

To improve digestion and elimination, break up gas, and stop intestinal spasms, physicians look to foods and supplements that contain:

- Chamomile
- Fennel
- Ginger
- Peppermint
- Rosemary
- Thyme

Water thyself!

Think of a great green lawn with an abundant garden. What does it require to stay healthy? <u>Frequent watering</u>. It's the same for our colon. Water helps cleanse the colon and lubricate the bowel that speeds up the elimination. <u>The new rule of thumb is to drink half your body weight in ounces.</u> So if you weigh 150 pounds, drink 75 ounces of water daily.

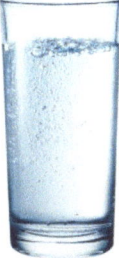

A Special Note on Children

Children's constipation can frequently be cleared up by adding more fibrous foods to their diets, making sure they exercise, and by giving them sufficient time for bathroom breaks. "Parents often don't give their children enough time to go every day; they rush them in the morning and don't give them fifteen minutes to just sit there. They don't have time to go so they just hold it," says Deborah Wiancek, N.D. of the Riverwalk Natural Health Clinic in Colorado: "When I ask kids about this and they tell me they aren't having bowel movements every day, the parents are surprised because they never ask, it's not part of their conversation," says Wiancek.

Sadly, this isn't something you'll find discussed at a medical doctor's office either. As Wiancek explains:

"When you go to a regular medical doctor, they usually don't even ask the question. The constipation can result in dysbiosis, which is an imbalance of intestinal flora and fauna (good and bad bacteria); and a reabsorption of metabolic and dietary toxins, including unstable forms of hormones and gastrointestinal complaints and systems. Plus, kids that are constipated often suffer from hemorrhoids. Food can get lodged in the large intestines near the appendix on the right side of the abdomen and it can inflame and rupture. "Bottom line is kids are simply not eating healthy. Instead, they're eating more processed and convenience food and foods with preservatives and additives. Fast food means white flour, red meat, saturated fats, and sugar. They all definitely contribute to constipation."

To encourage children to enjoy a wide variety of foods, begin when they are infants. Researchers found that children who were repeatedly offered unfamiliar, or disliked foods, increased their acceptance of them anyway. The key is to keep loads of healthy foods in the house; so no matter what's eaten, it's a nutritional win. A study by American Dietetic Association shows that mothers who eat lots of fruits and vegetables have children who are less likely to be "picky eaters;" and make sure to have that ever-important water handy so kids can reach for it often.

YOUR NOTES

CHAPTER FOUR

A PINCH OF THIS, A PINCH OF THAT

"The shoe that fits one person pinches another; there is no recipe for living that suits all cases."

Carl Jung

Oh, but if we were only talking about shoes! What's put into our food from farm or dairy to table can be good or bad depending on the specific type of additive. Food additives perform many valuable functions like increasing flavor, adding extra minerals or other nutrients, and delaying spoiling. They may be naturally-occurring food substances such as vinegar (acetic acid). But you should not assume that additives (*even natural ones*) are always safe.

Most food additives go through intensive safety testing before the Food and Drug Administration (FDA) approves them for human consumption, but some additives have avoided scrutiny. In 1958 the FDA compiled a list of generally recognized as safe (GRAS) additives that weren't required to undergo testing yet *every additive in use before that year made it onto the list!* Estimates suggest that the average American consumes five to 10 pounds of dubious flavorings, preservatives, and dyes each year.

Although the federal government later removed some dangerous substances from the GRAS list, many additives of questionable safety still remain. They include:

- Acacia gum, also known as Gum Arabic, is generally found in chewing gum, candies, and frostings. Similar gums are Carrageenan, Gum tragacanth, and carob or lotus bean gum which appear in ice cream, jellies, salad dressings, baked goods, gelatin desserts, and beverages.
  <u>NOTE</u>: *Asthma, rashes, and abnormal embryo development are all possible effects of these vegetable gums.*

- Alginic acid (or Algin gum/derivatives) similar to Ammonium alginate, sodium alginate, and propylene glycol alginate appear in beverages, cheeses, frozen treats, icings, and salad dressings.
  <u>NOTE</u>: *The possible side effects are reproductive problems and birth defects. It has also caused fetal death in animals.*

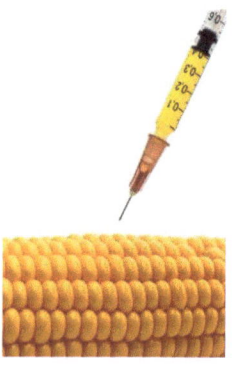

- Benzoic acid is also known as Sodium benzoate. It appears in baked goods, barbecue sauce, beverages, candy, gum, icings, margarine, and pickles.
  NOTE: Gastrointestinal irritation, asthma, rashes, irritation of the eyes and mucous membranes, neurological disorders, and hyperactivity in children are all possible effects from Benzoic acid or Sodium benzoate.

- BHA/BHT is found in baked goods, beverages, cereal, candy, rice, freeze-dried meats, potato flakes, soup, gelatin desserts, and ice cream.
  NOTE: Elevated cholesterol, allergic reactions, liver damage, kidney damage, infertility, vitamin D deficiency, and weakening of the immune system are all possible effects of this preservative.

- Iron salt is also known as ferrous lactate or ferric sodium pyrophosphate. Iron salts are found in grain-based products.
  NOTE: Gastrointestinal irritation and tumors are both possible effects.

- MSG is also known as glutamic acid hydrochloride, autolyzed yeast, yeast extract, hydrolyzed protein and hydrolyzed plant protein. Similar compounds are monoammonium and monopotassium glutamates. Glutamates are used as flavorings in baked goods, candy, condiments, Chinese food, pickles, sausages, soups, and sodium-free salt substitutes.
  NOTE: Possible effects are allergic reactions, facial and chest pressure, headaches, eye inflammation, high blood pressure, brain edema, depression, irritability, and central nervous and vascular system problems.

- Propylene gallate appears in baked goods, beverages, candy, gum, cereal, frozen treats, gelatin desserts, potato flakes, mayonnaise, and vegetable oils.
  NOTE: Possible effects are stomach and skin irritation, allergic reactions, liver and kidney damage. According to new research conducted at the University of Liverpool, nerve cells exposed to combinations of additives (such as MSG, aspartame, artificial colorings, in the amount found in typical snacks) experienced stunted growth and disrupted signaling.

- Food that lists *light, lite, diet,* or *low calorie* on the cover may contain aspartame (or Equal™ and NutraSweet™).

YOUR NOTES

CHAPTER FIVE

SUPER FOODS

"You don't have to cook fancy or complicated masterpieces - just good food from fresh ingredients."
Julia Child

Most of our lives we don't give a second thought to what we are eating unless we get sick. Then all those messages that lurk in the back of our brains emerge – tomatoes are good for you; tomatoes are bad for you. Look at what the Italians and Japanese eat or our Paleolithic ancestors ate. Try raw food only. Start juicing. Become a vegetarian or a vegan. Eat five small meals a day. Take supplements. Can you hear the voices in your head? *It is overwhelming!*

Science has come a long way in identifying what constitutes a 'good' food or a 'bad' food but what may be perfectly fine for you may be disastrous for someone else. In this book, I try to give an overview for a reasonably healthy person or one who wants to alter detrimental eating habits. Julia Child was right – "good food from fresh ingredients." From what I've spent my life learning, these are some of the best and why:

♀ BEST ♂

BERRIES
(Blueberries, cranberries, blackberries, Goji berries, raspberries & strawberries)

♀ WHY ♂

They are packed with disease fighting antioxidant compounds in the polyphenol family.

They contain some of the same healthy compounds found in red wine, but at 10 to 40 times the concentration.

Researchers also believe that fruit and vegetables rich in anthocyanins (the plant pigments that make blueberries blue and raspberries red) significantly reduce blood pressure and may have anti-inflammatory properties.

Research also indicates that anthocyanins may also improve vision, especially night vision, and eyestrain symptoms.

Although urinary tract infections (UTIs) can have a genetic component, one recent study showed that frequent consumption of any kind of berry juice correlated to a decreased risk of (UTI) reoccurrence. Cranberries in particular contain a special type of proanthocyanidin that prevents bacteria from sticking to the walls of the urinary tract.

Cranberries are also believed to prevent dental plaque, ulcers, and even heart disease.
The frequent consumption of blueberries enhances blood flow by increasing artery flexibility.

In addition to the antioxidant anthocyanins (which is three times the power of vitamin C), berries supply a wealth of phytochemicals, including flavonoids, caffeic acid, and elliagic acid, that protect against highly reactive oxidants that damage the brain.

Raspberries' elliagic acid helps to kill certain types of cancer cells, and black raspberries show promise in helping to prevent colon cancer.

Red raspberries are also believed to help ease child delivery, menstrual pain, and morning sickness. The Goji berry stimulates the release of human growth hormones and has been used for the treatment of insomnia.

Goji's betaine and polysaccharides can repair damaged DNA and enhance, or balance, the activity of all classes of immune cells.

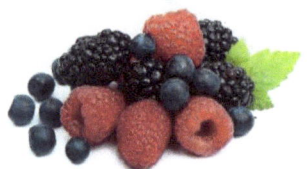

♀ BEST ♂

BANANAS

♀ WHY ♂

Compared to apples, they have twice the carbohydrates, 3 times the phosphorous, 4 times the protein, 5 times the vitamin A and Iron, and are also extremely rich in potassium, low pesticide levels, and are relatively inexpensive.

Potassium is a vital mineral, which helps normalize the heartbeat, sends oxygen to the brain, and regulates your body's water balance.

Bananas also contain tryptophan, a type of protein that the body converts into serotonin, known to make you relax and improve your mood and generally make you feel happier.

The banana is used against intestinal disorders because of its soft texture and smoothness. It is the only raw fruit that can be eaten without distress in over-chronicler cases.

It also neutralizes over-acidity and reduces irritation by coating the lining of the stomach.

The combination of vitamin A and potassium moisturize skin when applied externally.

GARLIC

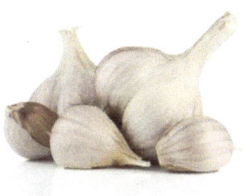

Garlic (Allium Sativum) and Wild Garlic (Allium Ursinum) has been shown to protect white and red blood cells from oxidative damage (caused by metals in the blood stream) and also has its own valid detoxification functions.

Garlic contains sulph-hydryl, which oxidizes mercury, cadmium, and lead and makes these metals water-soluble thus easier for the organism to excrete.

Garlic also contains alliin (which is enzymatically transformed into allicin), nature's most potent antimicrobial agent, which fights bacterial infection and possibly viruses.

Most selenium products are poorly absorbable and do not reach those body compartments in need of it. Garlic selenium is the most beneficial natural bio-available source.

The half-life of allicin (after crushing garlic) is less than 14 days. Most commercial garlic products have no allicin releasing potential left. This distinguishes freeze-dried garlic from all other products.

Garlic supplements might reduce cholesterol levels by inhibiting the activity of HMG-CoA reductase, an enzyme involved in cholesterol production.

Garlic is also a mild blood thinner and might slightly reduce blood pressure.

Garlic has also been believed to ease ear pain and dissolve mucus.

♀ BEST ♂

WATERMELON

♀ WHY ♂

Watermelon has 15 to 20 mg of lycopene in every two-cup serving; that's more than four times the amount found in a fresh medium-sized tomato.

23

Recent studies link high levels of lycopene in the blood with a lower cancer risk (especially prostate), heart disease, as well as a lower risk of macular degeneration. Varieties with yellow or light pink flesh may not deliver the optimum amount of lycopene.

Watermelon is an excellent source of vitamin A and B6.

There are 330 grams of potassium in two cups of watermelon.

Watermelon is also believed to have an alkalizing effect on the body.

♀ BEST ♂

ORANGE VEGETABLES

♀ WHY ♂

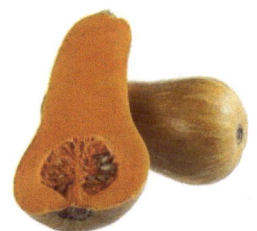

Pumpkins and winter squash are an excellent source of the antioxidant beta carotene, which the body turns into vitamin A. This maintains the health of cell membranes and boosts one's immunity.

Pumpkins and carrots come in a wide variety of colors from vivid red to yellow, and some pumpkin varieties are even white or gray. But only the orange varieties are a source for curative lutein, which is important for your eyes, skin, and heart.

To maximize the carotenoids' benefits, add a little fat to your carrots. For example, add a slice of avocado or black olives in a salad; or choose a salad dressing that contains olive oil. Also when snacking on baby carrots use organic low-fat yogurt dip.

Pumpkins are also high in vitamin E, fiber, potassium, and zinc.

♀ BEST ♂

BARLEY & ALFALFA

♀ WHY ♂

Barley is rich in fiber and is a good source for beta glucans, lignans, proteins, B-complex vitamins, vitamin E and a variety of minerals such as calcium, copper, iron, potassium, sulfur, and zinc.

Be sure to look for <u>hulled whole barley</u>! The polished, or pearl, barley found in supermarkets has had most of its fiber, protein, and vitamins refined away.

Before a kernel of barley has been formed, its grass is a concentrated source of amino acids, enzymes, vitamins, minerals, and healing phytochemicals. Research has shown that cereal grasses are a potent antidote to the toxic effects of dubious additives and synthetic insecticides.

Juiced barley grass is rich in chlorophyll, antioxidant enzymes, B and C vitamins, and a form of vitamin E-alphatocopherol succinate.

Alfalfa is similar in a lot of ways – it contains basically all the vitamins and minerals known to man, stimulates the pituitary gland, contains chlorophyll, alkalizes the body rapidly, and detoxifies the liver.

♀ **BEST** ♂

GREENS

♀ **WHY** ♂

Kelp may improve the conditions of thyroid disorders, cellular disease, connective tissue disorders, blood glucose levels, circulatory system, and high cholesterol. It is known to cleanse radiation from the body. It also contains iodine, sodium, and calcium. Kelp also provides nutritional support to the nervous system and heart.

Red Clover may improve the conditions of menopause, weak hormones, weak ovaries, cardiovascular disorders, high cholesterol, respiratory problems (bronchitis, asthma), skin disorders, (eczema, psoriasis), prostate abnormalities, muscle atrophy and it purifies the blood as well as relaxes the nerves.

Parsley is high in copper, vitamin B, potassium and like other leafy greens, parsley leaves are rich in chlorophyll, flavonoids, and vitamins, especially vitamin C. Constituents of parsley's essential oil are known to stimulate the uterus, increase urination, reduce inflammation of the urinary tract, and kill microbes. Globally, various cultures have recognized parsley's ability to clean the adrenals, promote digestion, treat gastrointestinal disorders, and prevent kidney/bladder stones, menstruation discomforts, menopause, asthma, jaundice, and bad breath.

Dandelion may aid liver, kidney, and gallbladder disorders, constipation, hemorrhoids, indigestion, eczema, edema, and diabetes.

Spinach, kale, and collard greens provide folic acid, vitamin C, beta carotene, as well as other carotenoids and luteins (promotes eye health).

OATS

Oats contain special antioxidant compounds that help lower cholesterol and prevent cardiovascular disease. They may also help reduce the risk for certain types of cancer, similar to the way that fruits and vegetables do.

A compound found in oats called beta-glucan not only helps neutrophils navigate to the site of an infection more quickly, it also enhances their ability to eliminate the bacteria they find there.

Oat groats, steel-cut, and old-fashioned are nutritionally superior oats to quick-cooking or instant oatmeal.

In addition to its fiber benefits, oats are also a good source of selenium, manganese, phosphorus, B1, magnesium, and protein.

PRICKLY PEAR

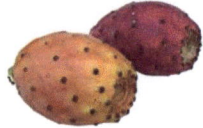

Prickly Pear (Nopal) is especially rich in vitamin C and contains easily digestible proteins.

Like aloe, it contains mucilage as well as pectin fiber. These contents support digestion and elimination.

A complex carbohydrate in Prickly Pear slows down the entry of both sugar and fat into the blood steam.

Prickly Pear contains various antioxidants that may curtail free radical damage to cell membranes.

Interesting results occurred when comparing the effects of Prickly Pear use between healthy people and those with diabetes. Prickly Pear significantly lowered the blood sugar levels of the diabetic patients, but not of the healthy subjects.

VINEGAR

♀ **WHY** ♂

Vinegar supplementation lowers glucose and insulin responses and increases safety after a bread meal in healthy subjects.

PRODUCE POINTERS

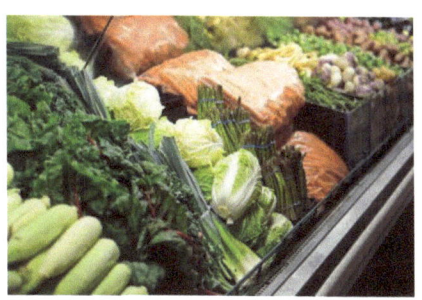

✓ When purchasing **<u>mushrooms</u>** look for dry and blemish-free tops. Store them in a paper bag in the refrigerator.

✓ When purchasing **<u>sweet potatoes</u>** you should look for smooth ones without any nicks or cuts. You can store them for two weeks in a cool, dry place. Do not refrigerate them; the temperature can create a hard core and an unpleasant taste.

✓ When purchasing **<u>peaches</u>** look for firmness with a slight give when squeezed and the fuzzier the fresher. Peaches will keep for 2 weeks in the refrigerator, or 2 days on the counter. Wash right before eating because the water breaks down the peaches especially fast.

✓ When purchasing **<u>pomegranates</u>** you should look for large red seeds that feel heavy for their size. They should have a wrinkle-free and crack-free skin. Pomegranates can be stored in your refrigerator for up to 3 months or three weeks at room temperature.

✓ When purchasing **<u>asparagus</u>** look for stalks that are all the same size to ensure equal cooking time and tightly closed tips. Wrap spear in plastic wrap in the refrigerator for 4 to 5 days. Before cooking, snap off the bottoms where they naturally break off. They're an excellent veggie for the grill.

✓ When purchasing **<u>dandelion greens</u>** look for small, tender leaves and roots are a definite plus. Refrigerate for up to 5 days in a re-sealable bag.

✓ When storing **<u>apples</u>** place them in a paper bag in the refrigerator or in a cool dark place for longer crisp periods.

✓ When purchasing **<u>watermelons</u>** look for an underside that is yellow or cream colored (if the rind shows any white, it isn't ripe), a melon that's especially heavy, and when tapped the melon it should have a low-pitched thud.

YOUR NOTES

CHAPTER SIX

MORE FOOD MUST-HAVES

"All you need is love. But a little chocolate now and then doesn't hurt."
Charles M. Schulz

Yes, chocolate! Good quality dark chocolate contains a large amount of antioxidants that protect your body from aging. Eating dark chocolate may lower your blood pressure and cholesterol while providing you with an energy boost. As I start providing even more information about the foods we need for optimum health, let's take a moment to salute our bodies and reward them with proper nourishment, including dark chocolate.

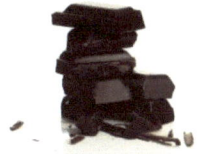

FATS AND OILS

Much of the information we learn about fats and oils seems contradictory and confusing.

- *Which fats are good for us?*
- *Which fats should we stay away from?*
- *What are lipids, triglycerides, fatty acids, saturated fats, and omega fatty acids?*
- *How do these relate to HDL and LDL?*

Fats and fatlike substances are called lipids. There are three major groups of lipids:

Phospholipids
Triglycerides
Cholesterol

Found in every cell, <u>lipids</u> are integrally involved in cell membrane structure, blood and tissue structure, enzyme reactions, memory, nervous system functions, vitamin D functions, the synthesis and the use of certain hormones, and hormone-like eicosanoids.

<u>Triglycerides</u> are what we commonly refer to as fat. They comprise 95% of the lipids in foods. Their principle function is as an energy source for metabolism, a function shared almost equally with carbohydrates. The excess calories we eat are converted to triglycerides and stored as body fat. Not only does this fat provide reserve fuel, it provides support and cushioning to the internal organs and serves as our insulation against body heat loss.

Cholesterol is found in all body tissue and is particularly concentrated in the liver, blood, and brain. The body supplies its own cholesterol (between 500mg and 1000mg each day) regardless, even if we do not eat cholesterol-laden foods.

Good Cholesterol versus Bad Cholesterol: Lipids interact with protein to form lipoproteins. These are small molecular packages of fat wrapped in protein. This allows the lipids to travel in the water-based blood stream. They are universally referred to by their acronyms: HDL, LDL, and VLDL.

Simply put, they indicate:
- ✓ High density lipoprotein (HDL, the good one)
- ✓ Low density (LDL, the bad cholesterol)
- ✓ Very low density (VLDL, very bad)

All of these forms are necessary for good health. But if unbalanced, they can cause health problems.

In the blood stream HDLs pick up cholesterol from dying cells and other sources and then are transported to the liver for excretion. The higher someone's HDL level is, the more cholesterol refuse is transported for dumping and the lower one's heart disease risk.

This bears repeating:

The higher someone's HDL level is, the more cholesterol refuse is transported for dumping and the lower one's heart disease risk.

Diets high in saturated fat will leave behind some LDLs and VLDL, which are scavenged by cells in the blood vessels where they become rancid and build up as plaque, narrowing the arteries.

The fat-free movement began with a scare around the saturated fats. Seemingly overnight butter, coconut oil, and palm oil disappeared from processed foods. They were replaced with hydrogenated and partially hydrogenated vegetable oils (which are also unhealthy), particularly from soy and cotton seed. People switched to polyunsaturated oils in cooking to lower cholesterol.

But then there was a connection between large amounts of polyunsaturated fats and cancer. After that we were saved by *olive, canola, and macadamia oil* that contain monounsaturated fats that lower LDLs and blood pressure and protect against heart disease. Just as proteins are made up of units called amino acids, fats are made up of units called fatty acids. The configuration of the fatty acids determines whether a fat is saturated or not.

The alpha and omega: The alpha is the carbon closest to the carbon group and the omega is the last carbon in the chain. Omega 3 and Omega 6 fatty acids are essential fatty acids that need to be included in the diet because the human metabolism cannot create them from other fatty acids. Excessive amounts of omega 6 polyunsaturated fatty acids and a very high omega 6/ low omega 3 ratio have been linked with many diseases. The ratio of omega 6 to omega 3 in modern diets is approximately 15:1, whereas 2:1 to 4:1 ratios have been associated with reduced mortality from cardiovascular disease and suppresses inflammation in patients with rheumatoid arthritis. A decreased risk of breast cancer is also a benefit.

CHAPTER SEVEN

FIBER - THE FIGHTER

"Part of the secret of success in life is to eat what you like and let the food fight it out inside."

Mark Twain

You are probably wondering why I am devoting an entire chapter to fiber. Mark Twain was partially right, as long as you consume the proper, nutritional foods. And fiber is the fighter – it *keeps the bad stuff moving on through.*

Although fiber has practically no nutritional value and is poorly digested by humans, it is still one of the best substances for humans to consume. More research has been done on fiber and its effects than almost any other nutrient essential for a healthy body. An adequate level of fiber is important, not just for the digestive system, but also to assist in offsetting a myriad of other potential health problems.

Consumption of dietary fibers can help lower blood cholesterol levels and regulate blood glucose and insulin levels, making fiber beneficial in the treatment of cardiovascular disease and can cut the risk of Type 2 Diabetes in half. In a ten year study of 68,000 women reported in The Journal of the American Medical Association it was demonstrated that eating adequate amounts of fiber lowers the risk of heart disease. However, dietary fiber intake continues to be at "less than recommended" levels in the United States. Part of the problem is public awareness.

When asked how much fiber they consume, 73% of American adults think the amount of fiber they eat is "about right." According to the American Dietary Association, most adults consume less than 15 grams of fiber daily, and yet the recommended intake for optimum health is 25 to 35 grams. Waste should be eliminated from the bowel within 24-36 hours after consumption, but for the average American adult waste is not eliminated for two to three and, in many cases, for five to six days. NOTE: Research from a comprehensive study completed in the 1970's shows extremely low rates of colon cancer among Africans who consume 10 times more fiber than the average American.

It is important to be aware that there are two kinds of fiber – soluble and insoluble.

> ▶ Soluble fiber helps slow the absorption of glucose from the intestines into the blood stream, and therefore improves the blood sugar balance as well as helping to lower cholesterol.

> ▶ Insoluble fiber causes more effective bowel movements and binds excessive fat and toxins in the digestive tract for elimination.

Daily doses of high quality fiber have been clinically proven to be beneficial in the following conditions:

- Lowers the risk of colon cancer.

- Assists in maintaining beneficial bacteria balance in the bowels.
- Reduces constipation.
- Helps prevent gallstones.
- Reduces cholesterol.
- Balances blood sugar levels.

The following are foods that are naturally high in fiber:

- Ground flax seed
- Beans
- Root vegetables
- Berries
- Peas
- Dried fruit
- Whole grains

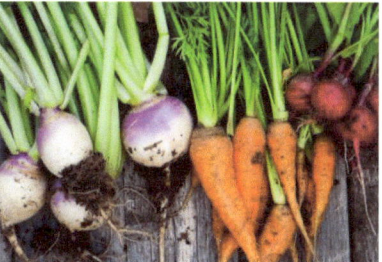

With there being such an increase of whole grain products, there has also been an increase of confusion over terminology, such as "whole grain" or "made with whole grain." Often such products contain a mix of whole and refined grains, two ingredients with opposite effects on health.

The European Journal of Clinical Nutrition examined diets and tested the blood of more than 800 people for triglycerides and cholesterol, and checked their blood pressure as well. The researchers concluded that eating whole grains decreased the risk of heart disease and diabetes, whereas eating refined grains increased these risks. Also two Harvard Studies found that adults who eat whole grains are less likely to be overweight.

When you're shopping you should look for "100% Whole grains or 100% whole wheat;" but I also find that checking the fiber content and reading the ingredients listings to be an effective way of determining if the grain has been minimally processed. Make sure to check for whole grains in organic products too, and don't let the presence of whole grains be used to encourage you into eating foods with sugar or saturated fat, like cookies for example. When increasing fiber intake it is critical that you drink plenty of water. Without enough water, the increase of your fiber intake could actually dehydrate your colon, cause gas, and sometimes constipation.

Psyllium vs. Flax

Many people that take a dietary fiber supplement use psyllium. What most people don't know is that most psyllium is imported from other countries whose regulation of pesticide use is more lax then United States. When the highly-regarded Consumers Union tested imported food for pesticide residues, they found that many contained relatively significant amounts of chemicals. In some cases, they found traces of pesticides that have already been banned in the United States.

Most Psyllium bought in the U.S. comes from India. According to The Financial Express, forty pesticides that have been taken off the market in most countries due to their deleterious health effects are still used in India. Indian farmers have access to more than 145 registered pesticides, but of all these only fifty have been studied enough to establish tolerance levels. Ravi Aggarwal, the head of Toxics Link in New Delhi told Financial Express: "All (Indian) government policies are pro-pesticides. It is the pesticide industry that is today the greatest deterrent to healthy farming. The extremely rich and powerful lobby of the pesticide industry controls government policies."

Ashutosh Halder Ph.D. with the All India Institute of Medical Sciences said "There is nothing called a safe pesticide. All of them are harmful. We need to demand that studies be done on how it affects health." Pesticides that have been strictly regulated or banned in the United States but widely used in India include:

- Lindane
- DDT
- Malathion
- Chlorpyrifos

Chlorpyrifos is a particularly troublesome pesticide. Research in the United States, shows that it causes severe birth defects. India's Central Insecticide Board reports that the country yearly applies 4,500 tons of Chlorpyrifos, the fourth most popular insecticide. *I will restate that most psyllium used in the United States is imported from India.*

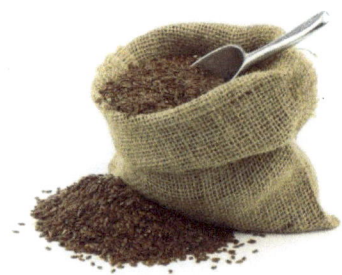

On the other hand, in a world full of toxins, organic fiber is a great alternative. Organic flax is certified and inspected as having been produced without the use of pesticides or other restricted chemicals. When you consume the recommended 25 to 35 grams of fiber through a diet rich in fruits, vegetables, and some grains you consume a ratio of 75% insoluble fiber and 25% soluble fiber.

Consider these facts:

- Flax provides roughly the same ratio of insoluble to soluble (75-65% to 25-35%), so it mimics the natural balance that a good diet provides.
- Psyllium husks provide the opposite balance of 20% insoluble to 80% soluble fiber.
- Psyllium absorbs water so effectively that it is used as a thickening agent in ice cream and as an additive to retain water in newly planted grass.
- Flax is also a useful aid to combat high cholesterol. In a study involving 40 patients with high cholesterol, daily consumption of 20 grams of ground flaxseed was compared to taking a statin drug. After 60 days, significant reductions were seen in total cholesterol, LDL, triglycerides, and HDL cholesterol in both groups. Those receiving flaxseed did just as well as those given a statin drug.

- Flax is also an excellent source of Omega 3 fatty-acids and lignans. Experts estimate that flax contains 100 times more lignans than any other source. Lignans enter the digestive tract and bind with toxins to help the body eliminate them before they can cause physiological difficulties. Lignans can engage with estrogen receptors sites in the body where the natural estrogen might otherwise raise your chances of developing cancer. Lignans also assist the immune system.
- Evidence of intestinal discomfort from the use of ground flax seed is hard to find, but complaints from the use of psyllium is apparently common.

In conclusion, flax seems to be the better choice.

YOUR NOTES

CHAPTER EIGHT

HERBS & SUPPLEMENTS

"Living in the ocean means never having to salt your food."

Takayuki Ikkaku

Why supplements? As the years have gone by, our food has moved away from nature; thus the increase in the availability of "natural" foods that create confusion since most – not all – are also processed and/or preserved in one form or another. If you work with a skilled practitioner, adding some of today's supplements (in pill, liquid, or crushed form) is highly beneficial for a balanced diet to replace what food processing and preserving has removed.

Enter our truly natural friends, the herbs. A USDA study reports that we can get far more antioxidants from herbs than from fruits and vegetables, including the grapes that are crushed to make red wine. A recent study from Norway has found that some herbs contain up to a 1,000 times more antioxidants than others. In this study it showed that the herbs found with the highest concentration of antioxidants were oregano, sage, peppermint, garden thyme, lemon balm, clove, allspice, and cinnamon along with a few Chinese herbs (Cinnamomi, cortex, and Scutellariae radix).

Other specific herbs to consider are:

- *Peppermint* is best known in breath mints and candy, but in herbal preparations and teas it is useful against a range of problems from digestion disorder to skin conditions. Peppermint offers antimicrobial effects against bacteria and fungi, helps reduce acute and chronic inflammation, and even appears to relieve menstrual cramps and toothaches. Peppermint is also believed to be an energizer and oxygenates the bloodstream. However, anyone with gastrointestinal reflux, hiatal hernia, or kidney stones should use caution with peppermint oil. Nor is this herb advised for people with gallbladder inflammation, liver damage, or bile duct obstruction.

- *Ginger* has been a culinary and medicinal favorite for the millennia. Traditionally used for dizziness, indigestion, nausea, and morning sickness, this spice has well-documented digestive and intestinal benefits. It contains one of nature's best proteolytic enzymes-zingibain, which is as effective as the papain in papaya and the bromelain in pineapple. Ginger contains at least 22 plant chemicals that effectively inhibit both 5-LO and COX-2, the enzymes most strongly implicated in joint inflammation. By stimulating bile secretion and fighting fat absorption, this spice can even help lower cholesterol levels. If you have a history of gallstones, do not take ginger.

- *Rosemary* is useful to combat arthritis, poor circulation, gallbladder disorders, indigestion, and pain. Cineole is an essential oil in rosemary that stimulates central nervous system.

- *Turmeric* generates enzyme secretions that help the liver detoxify dangerous substances in the body and has been used to treat gallbladder disorders hepatitis, indigestion, and pain relief. Turmeric may even halt cancer formation in breast and colon tissue.

- *Butter bur.* A randomized, double blind, study from Switzerland tested more than 300 allergy sufferers with butterbur herb extract, a popular antihistamine, and a placebo. Butterbur performed as well as the antihistamine and both were far more effective than the placebo.

- *Sage* has been believed to dry up breast milk, restore hair, expel worms, stop bleeding, and restore hair color.

- *St. John's Wort.* More than 18 million Americans will suffer from depression this year. Almost six million will take antidepressants. In dozens of studies, St. John's Wort has been proven to relieve depression of mild to moderate severity more successfully than a placebo and as successful as prescription antidepressants.

- *Cinnamon.* In Biblical times, this spice was used in holy oils and incense as well as in medicines and perfume. Today it is best known as a flavoring for foods and oral health products, where its antiseptic properties work to kill bacteria that cause gum disease and tooth decay. The hypoglycemic (blood sugar lowering) effects of cinnamon were discovered by accident when food scientists at the USDA found that eating apple pie had distinctly no dramatic effects on subject's blood sugars. Further study revealed that the cinnamon in the pie was to thank. As little as one-eighth teaspoon of cinnamon tripled insulin efficiency in USDA research.

  Cinnamon has been used as an aphrodisiac, circulatory stimulant, carminative (reduces gas), diuretic and digestive tonic. Today, cinnamon is listed as an herbal medicine for nausea, indigestion, and lack of appetite. Modern research has focused on its potential uses as an antioxidant, anti-inflammatory and cancer preventive. Much research has supported cinnamon's anticrobial potential. It slows the growth of fungi, including Candida yeast; and bacteria, including some strains of E coli and salmonella.

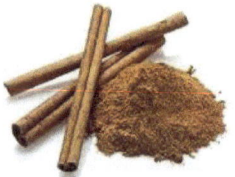

Cinnamon has garnered the most press, however, with its remarkable effects on blood sugar and insulin action effect that highlight the significant potential of this spice as an aid against Type 2 Diabetes and it precursor, metabolic syndrome. In 1986 about 30 million people worldwide had diabetes; as of 2006, that number has ballooned to 230 million. The U.S. government research is on the aromatic trail of cinnamon, hoping that this inexpensive and abundant spice will help to combat the serious worldwide issue of diabetes. Of the approximately 50 plant extracts tested, no others came close to affecting the metabolism of the sugars in the fat cells the way MCHP, a water soluble polyphenol in cinnamon, did.

NOTE: Cinnamon is very safe, but a handful of highly sensitive people may experience a mild allergic reaction.

- *Cayenne pepper* slows down bleeding (even arterial), improves circulation, heals ulcerated stomach, reduces fevers, helps to tolerate extreme temperature changes, relieves pain, aids digestion, and slows down gastrointestinal disorders and heartburn. Capsaicin (cayenne) alters the action of the bodily compound that transfers pain messages to the brain, thus reducing pain and inflammation. So, cayenne has become accepted as the active ingredient in over-the-counter and prescription creams (such as Zostrix) for post-operative surgery, cluster headaches, psoriasis and other skin conditions.

- *Tea tree oil* treats acne, athletes' foot, toenail infections, vaginal yeast infections, insect bites and stings, scabies and head lice. It's also used as a wound disinfectant and antiseptic mouth wash. Some believe it also is effective in sunburns, canker sores, poison oak or ivy, chicken pox, and ringworm. NOTE: Allergic reactions may occur and it should not be taken orally.

- *Aloe Vera.* Ancient Egyptian writings tell us that aloe vera has been used to heal humans for more than 3500 years. Roman records describe its use for many aliments including rashes, hemorrhoids, bruises, hair loss, tonsillitis, and gum and mouth problems. It was also used as an eye medication and helped to stop bleeding wounds. These applications are still typical today.

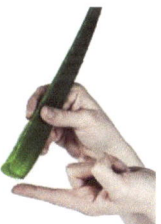

In the U.S. aloe is best known as a treatment for burns and sun burns; and as an internal cleanser and healer of the gastro-intestinal tract. Aloe is anti-inflammatory, anti-microbial, anti-histamine, and analgesic. Its beneficial mucilaginous quality brings alkalinity to a basically acid-eating population.

Studies since the 1930s have shown that the gel inside of the aloe's tough leaves speeds the healing of burns, wounds, frost bite, and a variety of skin problems (heat rash, dipper rash, poison ivy, hives, scabies, ringworm, athlete's foot exedra). Aloe also softens the skin and brings relief to dry skin.

Aloe stimulates the immune system, increasing white blood cell activity and the formation of T-cells. This helps to clear out pathogens. In addition, aloe reduces bleeding time, important to ruptured diverticula. A Harvard Medical School Book (2001) recommends aloe for functional dyspepsia, indigestion, and irritable bowel syndrome.

- *Essential oils.* Eucalyptus steam inhalations are effective treatment for coughs and bronchitis. Grape fruit, lemon, lime, and orange oils can be effective for relieving stress. Lavender, jasmine, rose, and ylang-ylang can have a relaxing effect. Bay, marjoram, oregano, rosemary, and thyme can fight infection. Wintergreen, peppermint, and spearmint can have a stimulating effect.

Other supplements that have beneficial effects include _Ginseng_ that affects one's energy levels, prostrate, insomnia, diabetes, depression and stimulates hormonal activity; _Echinacea_, a natural blood and lymph cleanser that also spurs mild antibiotic activity, increases T-cells, and stimulates immune response; _Burdock_ which is known as a blood purifier, diuretic, and may improve the condition of ulcers. It also helps move waste out of a weak body and expels kidney/bladder stones; _Chamomile_ helps one's nerves, toothaches, muscle pain, insomnia and helps normalize the appetite. It is also a gentle diuretic; _Horsetail_ helps slow hair loss, strengthens flimsy nails, move kidney stones, relieve skin conditions and aids in calcium absorption. It is also a diuretic.

YOUR NOTES

CHAPTER NINE

VITAMINS & MINERALS

"To all my little Hulkamaniacs, say your prayers, take your vitamins and you will never go wrong."

Hulk Hogan

As children, how many of us were told to take our vitamins! Mine was a brown liquid substance and I had to taste its icky thickness every night on a teaspoon before I went to bed. In as much as vitamins allow your body to grow and develop, they are also key to maintaining certain bodily functions. A proper vitamin balance helps improves your body's immunity, metabolism and digestion. Most vitamins can be acquired through food but some may need supplementation.

Vitamin C

Because humans can't manufacture or store vitamin C we need to consume it regularly; however Vitamin C is sensitive to heat and is lost in cooking water. The benefits of Vitamin C are numerous.

- Necessary for the formation of bones, teeth and cartilage
- Important in the healing of wounds, bruises, fractures, and capillary damage
- Prevents oxidative damage that leads to the development of disease
- Aids white blood cells that attack and destroy viruses, cancer cells, and other pathogens
- Enhances the immune system
- Is good for your heart
- Helps prevent high blood pressure and atherosclerosis
- Helps reduce the oxidation of LDL cholesterol
- Promotes healthy skin, joints, vision, and thinking skills

Vitamin D

For years, vitamin D deficiency was only identified with weak bones, muscle pain, and muscle weakness. Now there is mounting evidence that insufficient vitamin D is intrinsically linked to degenerative disease.

There is evidence that adequate amounts of vitamin D protect us against cancer, heart disease, diabetes, osteoporosis, autoimmune disease, periodontal disease, and some mental illnesses. In addition, deficiency has been linked to Crohn's disease and hearing loss while supplementations may treat the skin disorders psoriasis and scleroderma.

Research indicates vitamin D helps maintain healthy immunity and helps regulate cell growth and differentiation. It is called the "sunshine vitamin" because it is made in the body from an interaction between the sun's ultra violet B radiation (UV-B) and undeveloped cholesterol molecules in our skin. The body stores some of this vitamin D material as calcidiol, transforming it into the steroid hormone calcitriol. It signals the genes to make hundreds of enzymes and proteins crucial to maintaining health and fighting disease.

Exposure to UVB is essential – no sunshine no calcitriol. The best known biologic role of vitamin D is the maintenance of normal blood levels of calcium and phosphorus. When there is not sufficient vitamin D, the bones cannot lay down calcium. Vitamin D deficiency disease, also known as rickets in children and osteomalacia in adults, causes skeletal deformities (spinal curvature, bowed legs). The adult version also results in weak bones, global bone pain, muscle weakness, and muscle pain. The symptoms of osteomalacia are often misdiagnosed. One common disguise is fibromyalgia.

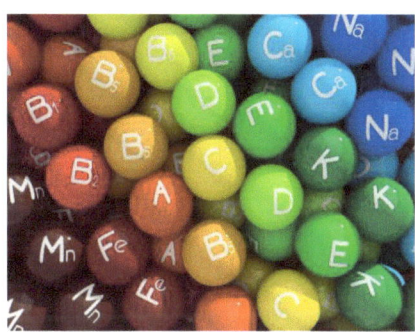

Calcium, Vitamin D & Disease

It is estimated that over 25 million American adults have, or are at risk of developing, **osteoporosis**. This disease is associated with low calcium intake. However, if there is not enough stored vitamin D, calcium absorption will be reduced. Meanwhile, we have become convinced that sunshine is bad for us. Some of us go for days, weeks, and even months without the sun touching our skin. Our bodies have no opportunity to synthesize vitamin D naturally, so as a result our vitamin D steroid hormone system is breaking down.

High blood pressure, another heart disease risk factor, is associated with problems in metabolizing calcium and with low levels of stored vitamin D. African Americans have a significantly higher prevalence of high blood pressure and lower vitamin D levels. One reason for this is that African Americans have an inherent difficulty accumulating vitamin D from sunlight. However, both short term daily supplementation with vitamin D and six weeks of UV-B exposure resulted in a reduction in blood pressure levels.

After years of being warned to avoid the sun because of **skin cancer** risk, vitamin D researchers are pointing out that the possibility of dying from low vitamin D status is far greater than that of dying from UV induced skin cancers. A 3 year study of 3,000 adults showed there was a significantly lower risk of advanced cancer lesions among those with the highest vitamin D intake.

At the 97th annual meeting of the American Association for Cancer Research, scientists announced that women who had greater exposure to sunlight during adolescence, or have high intakes of Vitamin D as an adult, are less likely to develop **breast cancer**. There were two studies that were offered at this meeting on this subject. The first was by the University of California, Santiago and it showed that a daily intake of about 1000 international units (IU) of Vitamin D was associated with a 50 % reduction in breast cancer risk. The current recommended daily intake in the U.S. is only 400. The second study presented by the Samuel Lynnfield Research Institute at Mount

Sinai Hospital in Toronto, stated that women who have the greatest intake of Vitamin D between ages 10 and 29 are predicted to reduce their risk of breast cancer by 40% .

It has been known for many years that normal insulin secretion depends on the presence of vitamin D. Studies show that low vitamin D activity delivers an increase in insulin resistance and reduced insulin secretions. A research group from New Zealand revealed that **Type 2 diabetes** is four times more likely in Caucasian Americans with low vitamin D levels (<18mcg/ml) than in those with higher levels (>32).

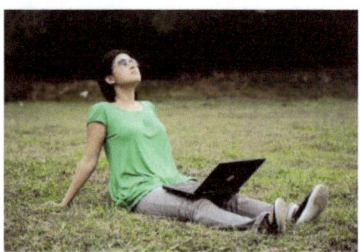

Keep in mind that if you have a dark complexion there can be a greater than 50% reduction in the amount of sun penetration you get in the same period of time as someone with a light complexion. In addition, a sunscreen with an SFF 8 reduces sun penetration by 97 percent. This does not mean we should seek a deep tan or burn your skin by overexposure. Overexposure remains a major cause of about 1.3 million new cases of skin cancer each year. The ultimate recommendation is exposure between 10 a.m. and 2 p.m. a couple of times a week with the time adjusted for pigmentation. Once you've captured the rays, then apply sunscreen. Delay showering an hour after exposure to give your body the opportunity to fully absorb the sunny vitamin D enhanced skin oils. The body has self-limiting mechanisms to protect it from manufacturing to much D from sunlight.

Vitamin A helps form and maintain healthy gums, teeth, skin, bones, and nerves and also supports good vision.

Vitamin B1 (Thiamine) helps convert carbohydrates into energy, and is essential for a healthy heart and nerves.

Vitamin B2 (Riboflavin) supports general growth and helps produce red blood cells.

Vitamin B3 (Niacin) helps maintain healthy skin, nerves and may have cholesterol-lowering effects.

Vitamin B5 (Pantothenic acid) is the "anti-stress" vitamin helps produce adrenal hormones and convert fats, carbohydrates, and proteins into energy.

Vitamin B6 (Pyridoxine) helps the body use protein from red blood cells and maintains normal brain functions.

Vitamin B 12 helps form red blood cells and maintains a healthy central nervous system.

Vitamin E is a potent antioxidant; a family of nutrients, not just a single compound.

Biotin (Vitamin H) is essential for healthy hair, nails and skin.

Vitamin K is the "clotting vitamin" and helps maintain strong bones in the elderly.

Folic Acid works with vitamin B12 to produce healthy red blood cells.

Vitamin K2 activates at least three proteins involved in bone health, and is effective in preventing bone fracture.

MINERALS

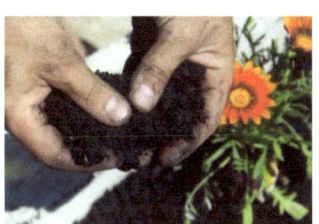

Calcium is good for bones, teeth, blood, and helps alleviate muscle contractions.

Phosphorus regulates the acid-base balance and helps forms strong bones and teeth.

Magnesium balances calcium, relaxes muscles, and is required for 350 enzymes to function.

Sodium balances fluids and blood pressure and is necessary for muscle function.

Potassium balances fluids and helps lower blood pressure.

Chloride balances fluids and aids digestion.

Sulfur is necessary for healthy hair, skin and nails, and essential for hormone production.

Iron is a component of hemoglobin and its enzymes help transport oxygen.

Iodine is part of the thyroid hormones, prevents goiter, and may reduce breast cancer cells.

Zinc strengthens immunity, aids wound healing and blood clotting, and delays macular degeneration.

Copper makes red blood cells and aids iron metabolism.

Manganese strengthens bones, helps produce collagen, and metabolizes cholesterol and carbohydrates.

Chromium maintains normal levels of blood glucose to help prevent diabetes.

YOUR NOTES

CHAPTER TEN

SWEETS FOR THE SWEET

"I prefer to regard a dessert as I would imagine the perfect woman: Subtle, a little bittersweet, not blowsy and extrovert. Delicately made up, not highly rouged. Holding back, not exposing everything and, of course, with a flavor that lasts."

Graham Kerr

Within the last 300 years the average American's sugar intake has increased 4000 per cent. Consumption has increased from about four pounds of sugar annually to the amazing amount of 153 pounds per person per year, which is equivalent to over half a cup a day (this figure doesn't even include the amount of sugar substitutes).

The average teenage boy eats twice as much sugar as any other age or sex group. Some behavior modification classes reward children with candy when they have finished an assignment or have not disturbed the class. Sweets' influence on American culture is alarming from Girl Scout Cookies™, to church bake sales, to birthday cakes; and the list goes on and on.

There is plenty of information on sugar and children. The problem is that it is so "controversial." Some research shows that it does cause hyperactivity and aggressiveness in children. Other research shows that it does not seem to cause any abnormal behavior. Three university behavioral researchers evaluated the diet changes instituted during 1980 to 1983 by Dr. Elizabeth Cagan, of the New York Public School System. After there were major dietary policy revisions involving sucrose, fats, and food additives, the schools showed a significant rise in national percentile ranking based on achievement test scores that correlated to the percentage of children eating school food. Before the diet changes, the 804 schools averaged in the 41 percentile nationally (1976-79).

Thus, during the four years in which the diet changes occurred, the mean national academic performances ranking rose to a 51 percentile. New York City schools moved from 11% below the national average to 5% above the national mean average. When sugar is removed from the child's diet miraculous things happen because children's bodies regain health easily when substances are removed that have been upsetting their body chemistry.

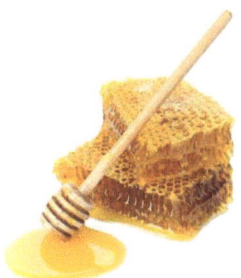

Therefore, instead of refined white sugar, physicians and scientists recommend the following substitutes:

Lo Han Extract
Raw Honey
Blackstrap Molasses
Brown Rice Syrup
Barley Malt
Date Sugar
Yacon
Stevia
Agave Syrup

Lo Han Kuo extracts are produced from both dried and fresh fruit. The extracts contain 80% or greater Mogroside. Mogroside is 300 times sweeter than cane sugar and is low in calories. It is a stable, non-fermentable extract which is ideal for diabetics.

Raw honey reportedly has medicinal benefits and contains enzymes and very small amounts of minerals and B-complex vitamins. Honey should not be given to children under the age of 18 months because their digestive tracts and immune systems are not yet developed enough for bacteria that may be present in honey. Honey varies in composition and flavor, depending on the source of the nectar (clover, orange blossom, sage, etc.). Honey contains about 38% fructose, 31% glucose, 1% sucrose, 9% other sugars, 17% water and 0.17% ash. Commercial honey is heated to 150 to 160°F, "Organic" or "raw" honey has not been heat-treated. Darker honeys contain higher amounts of minerals than lighter honeys.

Blackstrap molasses is the final product produced in the sugar-making process. As the final product, blackstrap molasses contains more vitamins, minerals, and trace elements (iron, potassium, calcium, copper, manganese, B6 vitamin, selenium, and magnesium) found naturally in the sugar cane plant, making it more nutritious than most other sweeteners. Traditionally, sugar cane processing involves three boiling processes to extract the juice. The first, boiling, produces light molasses; the second, dark molasses; and third, blackstrap molasses. Avoid the molasses usually found in the supermarket that blend the molasses with a sugar solution to ensure uniform quality. Barbados molasses is lighter and sweeter than blackstrap because it has higher sucrose content than blackstrap. Choose the Barbados variety only when the blackstrap variety is too strong or not sweet enough.

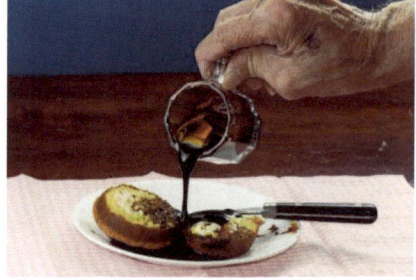

Brown rice syrup contains 50% soluble complex carbohydrates, which take from two to three hours to be digested, resulting in a steady supply of energy. This syrup can be evaporated to form a rice syrup powder. Brown rice syrup is a naturally processed sweetener made from sprouted brown rice. It is thick and mild-flavored.

Barley malt is made by fermenting grain. The fermenting bacteria convert the grain starches into simple and complex sugars and the final product consists of 40% complex carbohydrates. Barley malt is a thick, dark, slow-digesting sweetener made from sprouted barley. Malted barley has a high complement of enzymes for converting its starch supply into simple sugars. It also contains protein which is needed for yeast nutrition. Barley malt extract (available in powder and liquid forms) is also used medicinally as a bulking agent to promote bowel regularity.

Date sugar is made by pulverizing dried dates. It is not "refined" like sugar and therefore contains the nutrients and minerals found in dates. Date sugar also contains fiber.

Yacon root is a tasty root that scientists say is good for the gut, potentially safeguards against cancer, helps absorption of calcium and vitamins, and can reduce the blood sugar peaks from eating sweet food that make trouble for diabetics. Yacon has a crunchy texture like a water chestnut and is refreshingly sweet and juicy. It can be eaten as a fruit, consumed in drinks, or in syrups, cakes, or pickles. It's packed with the sugar, called oligofructose, which cannot be absorbed by the body. It also contains half the calories of sugar and promotes beneficial bacteria in the colon.

Stevia Rebaudiana is completely non-toxic, does not raise blood sugar levels, has no calories, and may help *prevent* cavities. It is much sweeter than sugar (10-15 times sweeter) and does not have the unhealthy disadvantages that you get with sugar. The refined extracts of Stevia (steviosides) may be 200-300 times sweeter than refined sugar. It has been used to sweeten foods and beverages for centuries. However, most of the nutritional benefits are minimal considering the small quantity that is typically consumed, especially concerning extracts since they are more refined. But unlike refined sugar, stevia won't drain the body of important nutrients and has an alkalizing effect on the body; though it does not caramelize like sugar does and some brands may have a distinct after-taste. Preliminary evidence suggests that it may lower blood pressure, prevent or reverse diabetes, and it possesses anti-viral properties.

Wild Agave syrup is juice extracted naturally from the core of living agave cactus plants. Similar to how a bee creates honey, it is through enzymatic action that the complex sugars in fresh agave juice are converted into simple sugars, producing agave nectar. The nectar is then finely filtered. The temperature in the entire process never exceeds 115°F. This minimal processing and minimal heat provides vitamins, minerals and enzymes in agave nectar that are not found in other processed sweeteners. Because of its low glycemic index agave nectar is suitable for people with diabetes and hyperglycemia. It absorbs slowly into the bloodstream, decreasing the highs and lows associated with sugar intake.

SWEETENERS TO AVOID

Common include:
- ✓ White sugar, pure sugar, granulated sugar, sugar, refined sugar, unrefined sugar, raw sugar, organic sugar, light/dark brown sugar, high fructose corn syrup, corn syrup, fructose, fructose corn syrup, dextrose, fruit juice concentrates, aspartame, sucralose, Equal®, Nutrasweet®, saccharin (Sweet'N Low®), powdered sugar, fondant, icing sugar, artificial maple syrup, glucose, fruitsource, Maltose, and Militol.

Less common include:
- ✓ Beet sugar, Turbiado sugar, inverted sugar, fruit syrup, isomalt, acesulfame k, neotame, maasdam, bottler's sugar, coarse sugar, manufacturers sugar, gel grain sugar, baker special sugar, liquicane type 50, corn stem/leaf fructose, corn stem/leaf sucrose, corn stem/leaf reducing sugar, corn stem/leaf non-reducing sugar, strawberry/watermelon/potato/peach/pea glucose, strawberry/watermelon/ potato/peach/pea fructose, strawberry/watermelon/potato/peach/pea sucrose, Ferricyanide Method, Ascorbic Acid Oxidase, and Sorbitol.

REASONS TO AVOID THE "EMPTY" CALORIE

Sugar and high fructose corn syrup are both highly processed sweeteners and offer no benefits to the health-conscious and environmentally responsible consumer. For some people there are disadvantages when consuming large amounts: increased LDL cholesterol levels, uric-acid levels in the blood, and triglyceride levels. Sugar's chemical name is *sucrose*.

Fructose (fruit sugar) is much sweeter than sucrose. The resulting high-fructose corn syrup is a liquid mixture of dextrose and fructose used by food manufacturers in soft drinks, canned fruits, jams and other foods. High fructose corn syrup contains 42, 55, 90 or 99% fructose.

The chemical makeup of sugar from a sugar beet and from sugar cane is identical. By the time sugar reaches the package or sugar bowl, it is 99.9% sucrose. For sugar cane, traditional processing involves:

a) Grinding the cane and pressing it to extract the juice;
b) Boiling the juice until it thickens and begins to crystallize;
c) Spinning and drying the crystals in a centrifuge to produce raw sugar;
d) Shipping the raw sugar to a refinery where it is…
e) Washed and filtered to remove the last remaining plant materials and color; and
f) Crystallized, dried and packaged.

Sugar adds calories and if you eat more than you need, you will gain weight. Weight gain increases your risk of getting heart disease, diabetes, high blood pressure, or even some types of cancer. If your body doesn't make enough insulin, like a diabetic, then the sugar you eat increases the sugar in your blood to unhealthy levels. The body breaks down sugar into glucose (the sugar you find in your blood). There are no vitamins or minerals in sugar and so it is called an "empty" calorie.

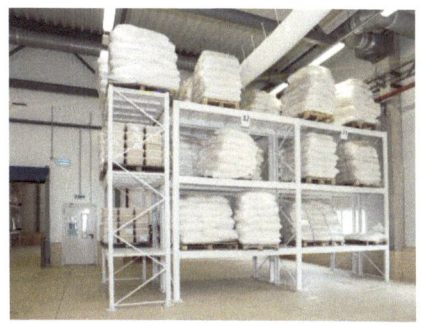

MORE SWEETENERS TO THINK ABOUT

Artificial sweeteners (e.g. aspartame) are among the food additives that have been shown to trigger hives, migraines, and people who are sensitive to MSG may also react to aspartame. *Saccharin* is made from petroleum and toluene, this sugar substitute is intensely sweet, calorie free, and linked to bladder cancer. *Sorbitol* is derived from corn, but sorbitol is more slowly digested so is used in diabetic foods. The benefit of sorbitol is that it does not promote tooth decay, however it can cause diarrhea.

Saccharin (Sweet'N Low®) Three scientific experiments in the early 1970s suggested that saccharin might be a carcinogen (cancer-causing substance) when given to rats in large doses. In response, the FDA proposed a ban on saccharin for all uses except as an over-the-counter drug. Significant public opposition to the FDA ban on saccharin ensued, prompting the FDA to pass the Saccharin Study and Labeling Act in 1977, which placed a two-year moratorium on any ban of the sweetener until further research was available. The law also required that any foods containing saccharin must carry a label that reads, "Use of this product may be hazardous to your health." On December 15, 2000, Congress passed legislation to remove the warning label that had been required on saccharin-sweetened foods and beverages since 1977.

Brown sugar consists of sugar crystals coated in molasses syrup with natural flavor and color. Many sugar refiners produce brown sugar by boiling a special molasses syrup until brown sugar crystals form. A centrifuge spins the crystals dry. Some of the syrup remains giving the sugar its brown color and molasses flavor. Other manufacturers produce brown sugar by blending special molasses syrup with white sugar crystals. The amount of molasses in brown sugar is so low it doesn't contribute enough of any vitamin or mineral to count on a food label.

Unrefined sugar is made from sugar cane juice that is released by pressing sugar cane stalks. It is different from refined sugar in that it is typically 50% less processed and therefore contains slightly more molasses than refined sugar. Unrefined sugar has a sucrose level in the range of 99.2% to 99.5% as compared to refined sugar which has a higher sucrose level of 99.9%.

Raw sugar is an intermediate product in cane sugar production. Produced at a sugar cane mill, it is a tan, coarse granulated product obtained from the evaporation of clarified sugar cane juice. The raw sugar producer ships this product to a refinery for final processing. <u>Consumers cannot buy raw sugar</u> even though it is high in sucrose - about 98%. The U.S. Food and Drug Administration says that raw sugar generally is "unfit for direct use as food or as a food ingredient" because it requires additional purification. The name brand Sugar In The Raw® is actually turbinado sugar.

Turbinado sugar is raw sugar that has been refined to a light tan color by washing in a centrifuge to remove surface molasses. In total sucrose content, turbinado is closer to refined sugar than to raw sugar (98% sucrose). As with brown sugar, products called turbinado sugar can be produced by blending white sugar with molasses.

Dextrose, a sweetener derived from corn, cane, or beet sugar to form a white granulated blend, is added by manufacturers and it may be less expensive than traditional sugar.

Fruit juice concentrates are highly refined sources of sugar that contain very little of the nutrients present in fresh fruit and none of the fiber that balances blood sugar. These sweeteners bear little resemblance to the fruit from which they are derived. It is recommended to use fruit juice instead of juice concentrates or fruit syrups, which are even more concentrated. A derivative of grapes is a highly refined product that usually contains about 68% soluble sugars. Food manufacturers use fruit juice concentrates as sweeteners. These fruit juices are concentrated through heat and enzyme treatments and filtration, which remove fiber, flavor, impurities and nutrients. A juice sweetener is essentially <u>identical</u> in calories, sugars, and nutrients to <u>sugar syrup</u>.

FOR SOME SWEETENERS, PROFESSIONALS ARE UNDECIDED, TOO

Sucanat ● Erythritol ● Barley malt ● Amasake ● Evaporated cane juice ● Splenda® ● Demerara Maple syrup ● Malt syrup ● Maple sugar ● Cinchona ● Xylitol ● Quinine ● Amazake ● Thaumatin

Sucanat is the only sugar cane product of its kind, is made by keeping together the two products that typical sugar processing tries to separate - sugar and molasses. Unlike brown sugar where molasses is simply added back to sugar for color, the molasses and sugar are kept together from the beginning of the process. This creates a dry sweetener product with the vitamins, minerals, and trace elements of the sugar cane plant and a lower sucrose level than refined white and brown sugar. Secondly, the crystals that are formed are actually bonded naturally, forming a granule that is easier to blend with the other ingredients and that creates a smoother texture in baked goods.

Erythritol or Eridex is the world's first all-natural non-caloric bulk sweetener and manufactured using a fermentation process. Erythritol occurs naturally in many fruits and vegetables.

Amasake is a traditional Japanese product made by fermenting sweet brown rice into a thick liquid. It is a creamy, quickly digested beverage used by athletes after a workout or as a sweetener in cooking or baking.

Evaporated cane juice retains more of the character of the juice from which they are recovered than the multiple-crystallization sugars. Although distinct colors, aromas, and flavors distinguish various sugar products, processing maintains the integrity of the sucrose molecule. Evaporated cane juice also contains a fair amount of riboflavin and small amounts of the vitamins, minerals, and trace elements found in molasses.

Demerara sugar is a popular product for tea and coffee in England, Australia, and Canada, but it is not very well known in the United States. It is often described as natural, unrefined cane sugar, and is light brown with large, slightly sticky crystals.

Maple syrup is made from the boiled sap of sugar maple trees. The taste and color vary depending on the temperature at which the sap was boiled and how long the sap was cooked. Maple syrup is a good source for magnesium and zinc. USDA Grade A maple syrup is the most popular grade for everyday use. It is usually made throughout most of the short syrup production season. Grade B syrup is generally made toward the end of the season. USDA Grade B syrup is much darker and has a stronger flavor, which makes it more suitable for flavoring and cooking purposes. It is thought that this late season syrup contains more minerals. Unless the product is labeled pure maple syrup, it is probably mostly corn syrup. *The real stuff is quite pricey.*

Malt syrup is yeast food and it gives products a pleasant taste, color, and aroma. There are two types: Enzyme-active (diastatic) and enzyme-inactive (nondiastatic). Triticale malts increase the levels of fermentable sugars and low-molecular-weight proteins in dough more significantly.

Splenda® is chemically processed as follows: Sucrose is tritylated with tritylchloride; this is performed in the presence of dimethylformamide and 4 - methylmorpholine. The tritylated sucrose is then acetylated with acetic anhydride.... The resulting TRISPA (6, 1', 6' - tri - O -trityl - penta - O - acetylsucrose) is then chlorinated with hydrogen chloride, in the presence of toluene. The resulting 4 - PAS (sucrose - penta-acetate) is then heated in the presence of methyl isobutyl ketone and acetic acid. The resulting mixture, 6 - PAS (sucrose -- 2, 3, 4, 3', and 4' penta-acetate) is again chlorinated with thionyl chloride, in the presence of benzyltriethylammoniumchloride and toluene. The resulting TOSPA (sucrose pena-acetate) is then treated with methanol; in the presence of sodium methoxide which produces the commercial product we call Splenda®.

Xylitol is a natural sweetener found in plants such as Birch trees, strawberries, plums, and pears; and is even produced by the human body during metabolism. Xylitol is actually a sugar alcohol because it has five carbons and five hydroxyl groups. Xylitol is similar to sucrose in its sweetness but has only 1/3 the amount of calories as sucrose. Xylitol is also absorbed slowly in the body and does not make blood glucose or insulin spike. But overall, the most widely discussed benefit of Xylitol includes its ability to be good for our teeth. Bacteria normally use sugar to grow, but bacteria can't use Xylitol and therefore Xylitol prevents cavities from forming. Xylitol also reduces plaque formation and increases salivary flow which helps clean and protect teeth. Adverse outcomes of Xylitol may be a slight laxative effect if it is consumed in large doses.

Thaumatin (brand name, Talin®) is a naturally-occurring combination of five sweet proteins derived from the berries of the West African Katemfe plant, also called the sweet prayer plant or the miracle plant. Thaumatin is metabolized by the body as a protein and has been found to be 3000 times sweeter than sucrose. It is not available in the United States, but it can be ordered online.

YOUR NOTES

CHAPTER ELEVEN

LET'S TALK ABOUT VEGETARIANISM

"I did not become a vegetarian for my health, I did it for the health of the chickens."

Isaac Bashevis Singer

It is the position of the American Dietetic Association and Dietitians of Canada that appropriately planned <u>vegetarian</u> diets are healthful, nutritionally adequate, and provide health benefits in the prevention and treatment of certain diseases. Approximately 2.5% of adults in the United States and 4% of adults in Canada follow vegetarian diets. A vegetarian diet is defined as one that does not include meat, fish, or fowl.

On the other hand, <u>fruitarians</u> avoid all animal products and processed foods. <u>Vegans</u> avoid all animal products. <u>Lacto-vegetarians</u> eat dairy products, but not eggs. <u>Lacto-ovo-vegetarians</u> eat both dairy products and eggs. <u>Semi-vegetarians</u> eat fish and/or chicken, but no red meat. They are not officially classed as vegetarians.

Interest in vegetarianism appears to be increasing, with many restaurants and college food services offering vegetarian meals routinely. Well-planned vegan and other types of vegetarian diets are appropriate for all stages of the life cycle, including during pregnancy, lactation, infancy, childhood, and adolescence. Vegetarian diets offer a number of nutritional benefits, including higher levels of fiber, magnesium, potassium, folate, antioxidants, vitamins and phytochemicals. Type 2 diabetes and high blood pressure occurs less often in vegetarians. No wonder that groups like the American Institute of Cancer Research, the American Heart Association, and the American Academy of Pediatrics today recommend a plant-based diet with a minimum of meat.

Moreover, people eating a plant-based diet also have lower cholesterol, body mass indexes, rates of death from ischemic heart disease, rates of hypertension, and risks of prostate and colon cancer than those whose diets that are not plant based. Prostate cancer is the leading cancer among men. In the year 2005 about 400,000 American men were diagnosed with it. A vegetarian diet can be a very healthy option, but it is important to ensure it is <u>well-balanced</u>. *You could easily stuff yourself with chips and chocolate at every meal and be vegetarian, but you wouldn't be doing your health any good.* Excellent food choices are whole grains, brown rice, legumes, nuts, seeds, fruit, vegetables, eggs, and yogurt.

YOUR NOTES

CHAPTER TWELVE

IS YOUR FOOD FAST OR JUNK?

"Just because the Americans are so good at rattling out accessible and cheap junk food, nobody looks twice when it comes to their food. But there are golden nuggets everywhere."

Jamie Oliver

At a pancake breakfast at church one Sunday, a young man brought our full plates so quickly I gasped with delight. He commented, dryly: "It's fast food." That was funny but the 'fast food' that is highly processed and that we buy at chain restaurants is not so funny.

Some fast food facts:

- In 1972, we spent $3 billion a year on fast food. Today we spend more than $110 billion.
- Each day, one in four Americans visits a fast food restaurant.
- The most popular hamburger chain represents 43% of the total U.S. fast food market.
- It also feeds more than 46 million people a day - more than the entire population of Spain.
- The burger chain operates more than 30,000 restaurants in more than 100 countries on six continents.

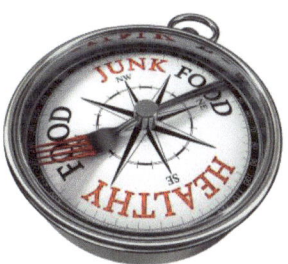

- Before most children can speak they can recognize a fast food restaurant.
- Americans eat almost 40% of our meals "out."
- French fries are the most eaten vegetable in America.
- A small order of fries was originally the only size - now their large size is 3 times that amount.
- In the U.S., we eat more than 1,000,000 animals an hour.

- You would have to walk for seven hours straight to burn off a super-sized burger, fries and soda.
- A premium ranch chicken salad with dressing contains >51g fat (79% of what is daily recommended)
- There are only seven items on a typical fast food menu that contain no sugar.
- On average if one eats 3 meals at a fast food burger chain, one will consume nearly one pound of sugar.

- One in every three children born in the year 2000 will develop diabetes in their lifetime

- If developed in your earlier years, diabetes can cut 17 to 27 years off your life.
- More than 60% of Americans get **no** form of exercise.
- 60% of all Americans are either overweight or obese, and America is the fattest nation in the world.
- Left unabated, obesity will surpass smoking as the leading cause of preventable death in America.
- The World Health Organization has declared obesity a global epidemic.
- The effects of caffeine and/or coffee can lower adrenal function, create adrenal burnout, lower thyroid function, create pituitary tumors/depress pituitary function, increase kidney problems, create iron deficiency, destroy the good bacteria in the gastro-intestinal tract, make our system too acidic, and impair digestion.

- If you are obese by the age of 13, there's an 83% chance you will be obese for the rest of your life.
- Elaborate coffee drinks can have as many as 800 calories per serving.
- A 12 year study of more than 155,000 women in the Nurses' Health Studies found that both regular and diet cola increased the risk of hypertension.
- In most homes the microwave gets more use than the stove top.
- The active ingredient in cola is phosphoric acid; its pH is 2.8 and it leaches calcium from bones.
- To carry cola syrup (the concentrate) the commercial truck must use the hazardous material place cards reserved for highly corrosive materials.

Of course, the choice is yours but, in my opinion, fast food may arrive quickly but it is not part of a truly healthy diet.

YOUR NOTES

BOOK ONE

SUMMARY

Since this is the first in a series of books in the **Your Health is Wealth**© collection, this summary may include extra information I haven't covered yet regarding the preceding topic matter. However, it will also give you an idea of how much more there is to learn about becoming the *Chief Executive Officer* of your own life-long health.

Therefore, in order to assess your own healthy gastrointestinal diet do's and don'ts, I've comprise a ranking system. I hope this will give you a sense of assessment concerning which changes will have the most influence on your health through diet.

The rankings run from easy to difficult with Beginner, Intermediate, Advanced, and Very Advanced. I assembled the ranking system in order to demonstrate that it is senseless to be concerned with minor issues, when you have yet to master the basics. For example you're wasting time and effort avoiding canned food (aluminum) unless you've kicked that diet soda habit. Don't get discouraged if you find advancing more difficult then what you estimated.

Being successful at "Beginner" is by far the most important and most dramatic achievement, and should be a treasured victory.

BEGINNER

Intensely Encouraged

- Eats more fruits and vegetables
- Drinks reverse osmosis water
- Adds unconventional proteins such as nuts, wild fish, and beans

Intensely Restricted

- Eliminates soda (including diet), sugar and all restricted sweeteners
- Excludes highly processed foods including hydronated oils, preservatives, and vegetable or grain-based snacks with less than 3gms of fiber
- Avoids animal meat products (unless organic or vegetarian fed, and hormone-antibiotic free)
- No fast food

INTERMEDIATE

Encouraged

- Includes organic produce (of the top 12 highest pesticide ranking and the top 4 GMO ranking)

- Drinks half body weight in ounces of reverse osmosis water daily (more with exercise, heat, or salt)
- Adds at least 25gms of fiber a day (beans, veggies, flax, and grains),
- Takes multi-vitamins

Restricted

- No canned foods,
- No psyllium-based fiber
- Does not cook or serve food with or on aluminum or plastic materials
- Does not frequent restaurants

ADVANCED

Encouraged

- Only fresh produce
- Ninety per cent of all food is organic
- Drinks reverse osmosis magnetized water
- Follows a ratio of 75% alkaline ash to 25% acidic ash (fruit and vegetables to grain, protein and dairy with few exceptions)

Restricted

- Does not use high heat or lengthy cooking times of produce
- Food and drinks are stored in inappropriate containers (plastics # 3, 6 and 7)
- Incorporates Juices with high measures of natural sweetness (unless diluted a third to a half with water)

VERY ADVANCED

Encouraged

- Vegetarianism
- All produce eaten uncooked
- Organically home grown fruits and vegetables consumed within 30 minutes of harvest
- Dissolvable multi-vitamins
- A 65% insoluble to 35% soluble fiber ratio
- Juices raw and homemade

FINAL THOUGHTS

Before you think that healthy choices aren't in your budget, consider how much of your groceries are instant pasta from a box or can, dinner mixes, potato chips, and carbonated soft drink, processed meats, frozen pizzas, ice cream, cookies, refined crackers with hydrogenated oils, imitation cheeses, or fast food (with a few exceptions) all of which are nutritionally worthless, but cost a lot of money and are unlike the vast nutrition that can be found in fruits, vegetables, nuts and legumes.

Another thing to consider with the financial decision is the cost of cold medicines, prescriptions, missed days of work due to illness, additional doctor visitations, or even surgery that could have been avoided if you had just decided to value your health enough to make it a priority – make your health your wealth.

I hope, in some way, that reading this book has improved your life and remember that knowing about an issue may not serve any benefit unless combined with determination to change. Thanks to everyone that assisted in the making of this book. Thanks for reading!

REFERENCE SOURCES

Royal Society of Medicine of Great Britain The Lancet, Minnesota Science Vol 54 no 1 2004, Decker Weiss NMD, Panela K. Hannaman-Pittman ND MS Dr. Theodore G. Aldhizer MD American Dietetic Association, American Medical Association 6/2/99, Diabetes Care 2004; 27: 538-46, Dr. Lindsey Duncan ND CN, US Surgeon General, American Chem. Soc Meeting 8/9/01, Nutrition Journal 2004 20:3 1:19, American Heart Association, Elaine Magee MPH RD, David Grotto RD, American Journal of Clinical Nutrition , Marco Falasca PhD

Financial Express 9/5/04, www.consumersunion.org, Ashutosh Halder PhD, The World Bank, Pak Tribune 9/9/03

Janis Jibrin RD, Ann Loise Gittlemen PhD CNN, University of California, Atherosclerosis 2004 173 2:2223-9 Journal of the American College of Nutrition 1993; 12:209-226, Lancet 1999 Aug 28 354(9180):740-741, Foods & Nutrition Encyclopedia, Life Science 1999;64(8):627-42

Deborah Wiancek ND, Decker Weiss NMD, American Journal of Clinical Nutrition, 1991 54:26IS-265S, American Dietetic Association, 2005 vol 105 no. 4, www.whfoods.com

Ann Louise Gittleman PhD CNN, European Urology 27: 104-109, University of Dundee, South Bank University, The National Cancer Institute, Professor Huffnagle, Earl Mindell RPH PhD, Farid Wassef RPh CNN, The Institute of Medicine, Related Metabolic Disorders 2004val 28 no7 Tokyo Imperial University, Archives of Dermatology (2006) 142: 615-618, Saengmurhak (July 2000) pp. 8-13, *Science* 6 (267): 90-931, *Nature* 22 (206): 757-761, The *Biochemistry Journal* 19: 339-339, *Science* 303 (5655): 186 – 195; Mayo Clinic USA Today (2001), John R. Lee MD, www.yalescor.org/past_seminars.html

www.wilsonsthyroidsyndrome.com/index.html, www.thyroidmanager.org, www.drrind.com, www.thyroid.about.com, www.thyroidpower.com/interadrenalthyroidfr.html

Harvard University Medical Journal, D. Eur. J. Cancer 27:131-5, Journal of Hum Ergol (1990) 19(1):53-62, Lancet (1999) 22; 353(9166):1742-5, "Dressed to Kill", www.selfstudycenter.org, Simon Cawthorne MD, Robert Mansel MD, Chronobiol Int (2000) Nov;17(6):783-93, Department of Environmental Health, Nara Women's University (Japan) Histol Histopathol (2000) Apr;15(2) :637-47, Clin J Pain 2000 Dec; 16 (4):298-303, Richard Santen MD, John McDougall MD, Michael Schacter MD, www.healthy.net, Theodore Potruch MD, Christiane Northrup MD, www.all-natural.com/fibrocys.html, Ralph L.Reed PhD

Natural Resources Defense Council, Nature (3/1005), www.nrdc.org, LiveScience (12/20/05), Lynn Keegan RN PhD, Gerald T Keegan MD, www.nsf.org/consumer/drinking_water, Sci Total Environ 11/1/05 and (11/25/05), University of Calgary, Cathy Ryan PhD, Joseph J Sweere DC, Environmental Working Group (2005), www.fda.gov, www.epa.gov, Clean Water Action Alliance of Massachusetts(12/04), Clean Water Fund, New York Times (12/4/04) Boston Globe (11/25/04) Sandra Stiengraber PhD, www.cleanwateraction.org,

Richard Loyd PhD, Mayo Clinic Diet Manual (3rd Edition), Herman Aihara "Acid and Alkaline" (5th edition), George Ohshawa Macrobiotic Foundation, "Nutrition Almanac 4th", Prescription for Nutritional Healing (3rd Edition), Dr. Otto Warburg, Elson Haas MD, www.energiseforlife.com/food_ph.php, New York Ballantine (p. 73-80), Hagiwara Yoshihide MD, www.aim4health.com/phind.htm Michael Colgan PhD CNN, Dr. Mary Ruth Swope, Yoshihide Hagiwara MD, www.rasnaturals.com/gettingstarted/acidalkalinechart.html, www.cancertutor.com

Dr. H. L. Bansel, Drs. G. Gerbenshchikow, Louis Donnet MD, Neuroscience Letter 1999 4;267:185-8, Society for Neuroscience (2002) Cancer Research 65, 8218-8223, (9/15/05) Dr. Michael I. Weintraub, International Journal of Neuroscience 1994 Jun Volume: 76 pg185- 225, Bioelectromagnetics (1996) 17:5, 358-63 Journal of Clinical Periodontology (1993) May;20(5):314-7 http://www.life-sources.com, Bioelectromagnetics 20(August):453, Journal of Neuroscience Research 55:230, American Journal of the Medical Sciences 316(September):176, Bioelectrochemistry and Bioenergetics 48(Feb):35.

www.saanendoah.com/ketosis.html, Gary D. Vogin MD, Rai Casey MD, Robert Sniadach DNH DC

Towers V "Users Guide to Healthy Digestion 2003, Robert Rountree MD, American Journal of Clinical Nutrition, Vol. 73, No. 2, 415S-420s, February 2001 www.energytimes.com, American Journal of Clinical Nutrition (1997) Vol 66, pp460-463, Journal of Nutrition 1989: 119, 112-115, Immunopharmacology 1997; 35; 229-235 CA Prima Publishing 1999:85-86, Phytotherapy Research, 1987;1:161-164

Royal Society of Medicine of Great Britain, The Lancet, Minnesota Science Vol 54 no 1 2004, Decker Weiss NMD, Panela K. Hannaman-Pittman ND MS Dr. Theodore G. Aldhizer MD

American Dietetic Association, American Medical Association6/2/99, Diabetes Care 2004; 27: 538-46, Dr. Lindsey Duncan ND CN, US Surgeon General, American Chem. Soc Meeting 8/9/01, Nutrition Journal 2004 20:3 1:19, American Heart Association, Elaine Magee MPH RD, David Grotto RD, American Journal of Clinical Nutrition , Marco Falasca PhD

Financial Express 9/5/04, www.consumersunion.org, Ashutosh Halder PhD, The World Bank, Pak Tribune 9/9/03

Janis Jibrin RD, Ann Loise Gittlemen PhD CNN, University of California, Atherosclerosis 2004   173 2:2223-9 Journal of the American College of Nutrition 1993; 12:209-226, Lancet 1999 Aug   28 354(9180):740-741, Foods & Nutrition Encyclopedia, Life Science 1999;64(8):627-42

Deborah Wiancek ND, Decker Weiss NMD, American Journal of Clinical Nutrition, 1991   54:26IS-265S, American Dietetic Association, 2005 vol 105 no. 4, www.whfoods.com

Ann Louise Gittleman PhD CNN, European Urology 27: 104-109, University of Dundee, South   Bank University, The National Cancer Institute, Professor Huffnagle, Earl Mindell RPH PhD,   Farid Wassef RPh CNN, The Institute of Medicine, Related Metabolic Disorders 2004val 28 no7

Tokyo Imperial University, Archives of Dermatology (2006) 142: 615-618, Saengmurhak (July 2000) pp. 8-13, *Science* 6 (267): 90-931, *Nature* 22 (206): 757-761, The *Biochemistry Journal* 19: 339-339, *Science* 303 (5655): 186 – 195

US Department of Agriculture, Amy B. Howell PhD, Arzneimittel-Forschung 1991 vol 41 no. 9, Journal of Biomedicine and Biotechnology 2004 no 5, Survey of Ophthalmology vol. 49 no 1, American Journal of Clinical Nutrition 2003 vol.77 no.3 Elizabeth Somer MA RD, Journal of Agriculture and Food Chemistry 2002 vol. 50 no. 10, Nutrition and Cancer 2001 vol. 40 no. 2,   Lindsey Duncan ND CN

Food and Drug Administration, Omer Kucuk MD FACN, www.watermelon.org, Joseph Levy PhD, www.urbanevt.uiuc.edu

Vincent Giampapa MD, Ronald Pero PhD, American Journal of Clinical Nutrition 8/04, www.foodnavigator.com

American Journal of Clinical Nutrition 11/04, Phyllis A. Balch, Elliot D. Abravanel MD, Eric F. W. Powell PhD ND, Journal of Nutrition 35:296-300, www.vrp.com, Lancet 1993; 342:1209-10, www.healthcentral.com, Nutrition Times Press 1994, www.findarticles.com/p/articles, John Heinerman PhD, J Ethnopharmacol (1997) 58(1):45-54, Acta Pharm Hung (1998) 68(3):150-56, HMA Scientific Committee 1996

Journal of Nutrition 2003 Feb 133(2):468-75, Foods & Nutrition Encyclopedia, *American Journal of Clinical Nutrition* 2004 Dec 80(6):1492-9, American Institute for Cancer Research Nov 3 2004, Foods & Nutriton Encyclopedia, www.whfoods.com

University of Texas at El Paso, Ray Sahelian MD, Journal of Health Care for the Poor and Underserved. 2004; 15(4):576-588, Archives of Latino Americano Nutrition 1998; 48(4):316-323

Diabetes Care (2004) 27; 281-282, European Journal of Clinic Nutrition (2005) 59: 983-988, European Journal of Clinic Nutrition (2005) 59: 1266-1271

US Department of Agriculture, Norwegian Crop Research Institute, Centers for Disease Control and Prevention, www.freedompressonline.com, Elliot D. Abravanel MD, User's Guide to Healthy Digestion

US Department of Agriculture, Alam Khan PhD, Bea Heller DC MS QME, Donald J. Graves PhD, James Duke PhD, User's Guide to Healthy Digestion
John E. Hahn DPM ND, Cichewicz RH PA, Journal of Ethnopharmacology (1996) 52(2):61-70, J Rheumatol, 1992; 19(4):604-7 Anesth Analg (1998)Mar 86(3):579-83. Elliot D. Abravanel MD

Robert Roundtree MD, Elliot D. Abravanel MD, www.Drugs.com; James Duke PhD, Raphael Kellman MD, Elizabeth Lipski MS RD LD, Dr. Dukes "The Green Pharmacy", Harvard Medical School Book 2001
Suzann Wang ND, Eileen D. Cristina CMP ACAD, Gary Young ND, Integrated Aromatic Medicine 2000, Isabelle Hutton RN

Journal of Agricultural and Food Chemistry 2003;51(16):4549-4553, European Journal of Herbal Medicine 1997;3:25-28, Public Health and Nutrition 2000;3(4A):473-485, Alan Bracer MD http://attra.ncat.org/attra-pub/echinacea.html, Coronary Artery Disease 2001;12(7):581-584, Annals of Internal Medicine 2002;137:939-946, Journal of Clinical Research 1998;1:367-380, www.cami.usip.edu/monographs/echinacea.htm, www.crop.cri.nz/psp/broadshe/burdock.htm, Oncology Report 2005;14(5):1345-1350, American Journal of Chinese Medicine 1996;24(2):127-137, Brazilian Dental Journal. 2005; 16(3):192-196

Journal of Clinical Pharmacy and Therapeutics 2002; 27(6):391-401, Biochemistry and Pharmacology 2000; 59(11):1387-1394, Life Sciences 2006; 78(8):856-861, www.mcp.edu/herbal/chamomile/chamomile, Sleep in Medicine Review 2000; 4(3):229-251 www.botanical.com/botanical/mgmh/mgmh.html, http://hgic.clemson.edu/factsheets/HGIC2301.html,

Jane Higdon PhD, American Journal of Clinical Nutrition 4/03, Shari Lieberman PhD CNS, American Journal of Clinical Nutrition 4/05 www.drrathresearch.org

John Cannell MD, National Institute of Health, National Cancer Institute, National Health and Nutrition Examination Survey, Iowa Women's Health Study
Journal of the American Medical Association (2002) 287;3116-26 3127-9, Vitamin K Laboratory at Tuffs University in Boston MA, American Journal of Epidemiology (2004) vol. 160 No 9 888-92, Carolyn Dean MD ND

Agriculture handbook No 8-4, Human nutrition Information Service, USDA, Barry Sears PHD, American Journal Public Health (1994) 84:722-724, Biomedical Pharmacotherapy (2002)56(8): 365-79, American Journal of Clinical Nutrition57(6):875-83, Biochemistry (2005) 22;44(11): 4458-65

www.betternutrition.com
Journal of American Dietetic Association (2003)103:748-765, Cyndi Reeser MPH RD LD, George Washington University Medical Center 2004, American Journal of Clinical Nutrition 1994;59 1248S-54S, Suzanne Havala MS RD, Mark Messina PhD RD, Victoria Harrison RD

Science 193:584, Economic Botany 9(2):108, Food Research 14:499, Journal of Agricultural and Food Chemistry 8:318, Journal of Food Science 35:769, Journal of Food Science 59: 197-205. Journal of Home Economics 58(6):479, Journal of Agricultural and Food Chemistry 5:773 Journal of Food Science 60: 405 h 9:462, Journal of Agricultural and Food Chemistry 3:346 http://food.oregonstate.edu/sugar, Advances In Food Research 3:241, Journal Of Agricultural And Food Chemistry 14:86, Journal Of Agricultural And Food Chemistry 11:230, Journal Of Nutrition 3:61,Food Production and Development 11(4):66, J. Food Sci. 40:784, The Sugar Association, Inc. Fast Facts About Sugar 1101 15th Street NW, Suite 600, Washington, DC 20005. 202/785-1122, Nancy Appleton PhD, http://www.nancyappleton.com, Goldman J. et. al, Behavioral Effects of Sucrose on Preschool Children, Journal of Abnormal Child Psychology 14 4 (1986): 565-577, Nutritional Behavior 1 (1984): 277-288. Nancy Appleton, Ph.D. Dr. William Crook, Foods & Nutrition Encyclopedia, Lancet 1980 Oct 11; 2(8198):809, Cancer Research 1995 Jun 1; 55 (11):2310-5, Cancer Research 1993 Sep 15; 53(18):4182-8

British Medical Association Dr. Arpad Pasztai, Columbia University, USDA, Richard Perez-Pena New York Times 3/22/04, Melissa Healy Los Angeles Times, Charles M. Benbrook PhD, Sandra Steingraber PhD, Denise Webb PhD RD, www.ota.com, Baillie Hamilton MD PhD, European Journal of clinical Nutrition, www.landinstitute.org, California Certified Organic Farmers, www.ccof.com, www.usda.gov/nass

USDA Meat and Poultry Hotline 1-888-674-6854 International   Dairy Foods Association, www.idaf.org, www.nopa.com, Center for Food Safety and Applied Nutrition (CFSAN), US Food and Drug Administration, www.cfan.fda.gov, USDA's National Organic Program, www.ams.govm, Organic Dairy Producers Alliance, www.usda.gov/nass, Union of Concerned Scientists, Warren Leon PhD, www.ucsusa.org, Karen Collins MS RD, Journal of the American Dietetic Association 6/03, www.seabear.com

http://www.supersizeme.com/home.aspx?page=bythelb Daryl Isaacs MD, Stephen Siegel MD, Bridget Bennett MS RD; Eating Patterns in America Boston Globe 10/12/05